Mountain Biking for Teens

Everything You Need to Know for Beginners

BJ Turner

contained within this document, including, but not limited to, errors, omissions, or inaccuracies.

Table of Contents

Introduction

Mountain biking is an incredible, adrenaline-filled sport, where you ride on all types of off-road trails. The sport includes many different cycling areas, from sand to forest, rocks, mountains, dirt roads, and even snow. Anytime a bicycle is on a 'natural' road, we call it mountain biking.

It is a sport that is loved by millions of people around the world, all cycling in their own unique areas. From the snowy mountains of Switzerland to the crazy-beautiful forests of South Africa, the trails of the world are never-ending.

Depending on what type of mountain biker you want to be, you need some level of skill to do mountain biking safely and smoothly. It is possible to get on a mountain bike and just ride without any training. But if you want to become a skilled rider. and learn all the tips and tricks of the sport, this is the right book for you.

As a long-time rider, I want to use this book to motivate other youngsters to try this sport, and understand why I enjoy mountain biking so much. Not only are you able to keep fit and healthy, but you are able to see some of the most beautiful parts of nature. And the best part, of course, is that you can use your bike to try new challenges and do things you've never been able to do before. I invite you to read this book if you want to learn about your mountain bike, or learn to ride skillfully. Thousands of cyclists ride every day, but some are still making silly or even dangerous mistakes because they don't know how to control their bikes well. In this book, you will learn to handle challenges that will make you look like a pro!

All you need to do is understand the skills we talk about in this book and practice, practice, practice. Everyone was a beginner at some point, even the professional cyclist. They also struggled in the beginning, and they couldn't always do the tricks they can do now. It's important to remember that. So when you are trying these new skills, and you are struggling to get it right, remember that everyone struggles in the beginning. And that's okay. The only way to stop struggling and stop falling is to keep trying until you get it right. Don't give up! It's not an easy sport, but when you get it right, it's worth it!

The History of the Bike

Bicycles have become such a normal part of our life, and we probably cannot imagine a life without them. Today, we don't just use bikes to travel, but we use bicycles to visit some of the most beautiful parts of nature, just for fun.

Before we look at what your bike looks like today, have you ever thought about what bikes looked like in the beginning, when they were first made? Bicycles have changed so much over the years, and you would not believe what they first looked like.

Before motorbikes, cars, and planes, bicycles and horses were the only way people could travel. As bicycles developed over the years and technology was added to the bike's design, we were able to do things with bikes that were never thought of! It's crazy to think that we have bikes today that have gears to help you ride better, when bikes didn't even have brakes when they were first designed!

The first type of bicycle was created over 200 years ago, and this type of bicycle was called a 'hobby-horse,' or sometimes they called it a 'running horse.' The crazy thing about these bicycles was that they had no pedals. To *ride* these hobby-horses, you had to sit on the seat, and use your legs to push yourself away from the ground.

A few years laters, a few inventors in France tried to make this design better by adding pedals, and this was finally called a bicycle. Through the years, the bike's design was changed in many ways. Designers tried to make one wheel extremely big, to help riders have some stability, but that only caused serious injuries when you fell off the bike. It was only 70 years after the hobby horse that someone designed the shape of the bike that we know today. They finally made both wheels the same size.

Since then, expert inventors and riders have changed the bike's shape, design, and technology, so that we have only the best types of bikes available today.

Chapter 1:

Choosing Your Type of Mountain

Bike

Finding the perfect mountain bike for you.

There are many mountain bikes available, and it can be tough to find the right one if you don't know what to look for. Choosing the right type of mountain bike will depend on what you want to be doing with your bike. Do you just want to ride on flat roads? Do you want to start doing downhill racing, or maybe do long-distance riding? Not all mountain bikes are the same, and there are a few differences between each bike that will make a big difference in how they ride.

Below are the different types of mountain bikes that you can choose from. Understanding each of these bikes will help you decide what you yourself should get for your mountain biking adventure.

Trail Bikes

Trail bikes are specifically made to take on the tricky trails you might find while mountain biking. They also make great first-time bikes, since they are built to handle just about everything. The main feature of a trail bike is the front part (known as the fork), which is quite hard. This is so that you have better control of the bike on tricky roads. These bikes also mainly come with dual-suspension, so that you can handle the difficult paths better (which you will learn about in the next chapter).

The main thing to remember about a trail bike is that they were designed to ride uphill and flat roads equally easily, and that they also ride happily on downhills. The bike's weight is also perfectly set if you need to do quick turns and ride uphill, without too much trouble.

Reasons You Should Buy a Trail Bike

If you want to try all kinds of mountain biking, whether uphills or downhills, this bike is perfect. You should also get this bike if you're unsure what you want to get, since it's great for all types of trails.

Reasons You Shouldn't Buy One

Do you know what kind of mountain biking you want to do yet? If you're going to do racing, like cross-country or even Enduro racing, this may not be the bike to get. It is not specifically made for speed, so you won't get the best results with downhill racing.

Cross Country Bikes

Cross-country bikes are usually for long-distance riding on pretty flat roads. They can ride uphill, and you will also get down a hill with this bike, but it wasn't specifically designed for that. Also, many of the cross-country bikes have a hard-tail (which means it doesn't bounce well on bumpy roads.) This can make it extremely uncomfortable on rough trails. Most trail bikes have suspensions, making it less uncomfortable when the rocky roads are shaking your bike around.

If you know that you don't want to be riding challenging trails, you can get yourself a cross-country bike. They don't have many parts that trail bikes have (like dual-suspension), because it isn't necessary on mainly flat roads. The main focus is the fact that they are light, even though they have some of the bigger-sized wheels. This makes cross-country bikes perfect for riding fast and riding long.

Reasons You Should Buy A Cross Country Bike

Get yourself a cross-country bike if you are looking to do races and don't mind if the bike is a little uncomfortable since it is a hard-tail after all. Having little suspension means you're in for a bumpy ride. If you enjoy racing long distances more than you enjoy tricky trails, these bikes are for you.

Reasons You Shouldn't Buy One

If you enjoy slower, comfortable rides, or want to ride challenging single-track trails, *don't* get yourself a cross-country bike.

Types of Cross-Country Biking Races

Cross-country biking is one of the most fun riding styles, but this also depends on what you like. If you participate in these types of biking experiences, here are some of the competitions you could join:

Cross Country Eliminator: These races are different distances, depending on the country and area. But usually, there are four riders competing at a time, and the last one to cross the finish line is eliminated from the race. These are also done in laps with someone eliminated each time.

Cross Country Marathon: These are some of the longer races where the distance is about 60 miles (100 kilometers) and combines all types of roads, from gravel to singletrack. These races usually have shorter distances for those who don't want to ride 60 miles, so you can enter the one that suits your fitness level.

Cross Country Olympics: Did you know that cross country riding is actually an Olympic sport? These races are like the racing they do in the Olympics, where the rules are simple. All the riders start at the same time, and have to finish a few laps around the course. These routes aren't very long and are sometimes only about 3 miles (5 kilometers) per lap. If your time is too far from the first person's time, then you are eliminated.

Fat Bikes

Fat bikes are a new type of bike that is made for riding on loose, soft ground, like snow or mud. Fat bikes are not actually *fat; it* is the tires that are big. These fat tires are great for riding on mud, snow, or sand because they have more control on the loose ground.

Best of all, because of the big tires, they can also roll over obstacles easily and can still ride uphill with no issues. So, these bikes are specifically made for uneven, soft roads, but it doesn't mean they can't ride on regular roads too.

If you stay in an area where it snows a lot, these bikes are a great choice.

Downhill Bikes

Downhill bikes are made specifically for downhill racing, so that the rider is more comfortable when moving the bike at such fast speeds. They make these bikes so that they are easier to control when riding down a hill and on rocky roads. This means that they weren't made for pedaling much.

Reasons You Should Buy a Downhill Bike

If you want to focus only on downhills, this is the perfect bike for you. It is made for speed and rocky trails.

Reasons You Shouldn't Buy One

If you are looking to do many different kinds of roads and trails, this is not the type of bike to get, especially if there are a lot of uphills. They are only for downhills, and will not help much on trails or hills.

Enduro Bikes

Enduro bikes are very specific for a very specific type of racing.

These bikes are basically the same as downhill bikes, but the main difference is they can climb hills slightly better than downhill bikes. That's because Enduro racing is all about racing downhill as quickly as you can. Of course, in order to get to the top of the hill, your bike has to get to the top. That's why it was built to climb as well. But with Enduro racing, the uphills are not timed, so most riders take it nice and slow.They are not as easy to control on trails as trail bikes, but they are able to roll over obstacles really easily on a downhill. And sometimes these Enduro competitions can go on for days, so the bike has to be designed to handle extreme riding.

Reasons You Should Buy An Enduro Bike

If you want to go down a hill as fast as possible, the Enduro-bikes were made specifically for that.

Reasons You Shouldn't Buy One

If you want to play around with your bike and ride different types of trails, an Enduro bike won't work for you. They can ride trails and do jumps, but the way they were designed makes it a bit more difficult to do.

The Difference Between Downhill and Enduro Racing

It sounds like downhilling and Enduro is the same thing then, right? But there are a few differences you can look out for.

Since Enduro is a specific type of race, where riders need specific skills, the bike is designed to work with those skills.

Downhilling: Downhill racing usually has one track that goes down a really steep hill or mountain, which is usually rough and rocky. The winner of the race is the person who can get down that singletrack in the shortest time. These races are usually only a few minutes, but the riders need a lot of energy and power to complete the race.

Enduro Racing: Enduro racing is also focused on downhill racing, but Enduro racing lasts a few days. There are usually a few different stages where the riders have to go down a few different rocky hills. The rider who has the best time down all the hills will then be the winner.

All-Mountain Bikes

All-mountain bikes were made to ride on a few different types of roads. They are made for riding smoothly downhill, and work extremely well on challenging trails. The tires on these bikes are a little wider, and the brakes are pretty strong, which is precisely what you need.

For beginners who don't know what type of mountain biking they want to do yet, these bikes are great as a first bike. They allow you to ride on all kinds of roads, and really get a feel for the sport. They are excellent at going down a hill, but also give you the power you need to go uphill, and can still move quickly on trails.

The main difference between these bikes and trail bikes is that they are better at going uphill, and they are experts at downhills.

Reasons You Should Buy an All-Mountain Bike

If you want to ride uphills comfortably and easily, and want to do well on the downhills, these bikes are great. They are hardy and strong, which is what you need on the uphills and downhills.

Reasons You Shouldn't Buy an All-Mountain Bike

If you want something light and easy that speeds on a downhill, this bike is not your first choice. Since it isn't very light and isn't built for speed, you won't have the same speed as with an Enduro bike.

Comparing MTB and Road Bikes

Mountain bikes and road bikes are entirely different. They are opposites in how the bike looks, how it rides, and where you can ride it.

The road bike frames and tires are very thin and smooth, and the seat is usually small. This is perfect for flat roads. But mountain bikes have much bigger tires, which are the best to stay stable on uneven, rocky routes. The seats are also much bigger and softer, protecting you from uncomfortable shaking and knocking against the saddle.

Both bikes have gears and breaks, but each works a little differently because of the different types of roads they can ride on. It makes sense that road bikes have fewer gears and their brakes aren't as powerful, since the roads they ride on are not as tricky.

Comparing MTB and BMX

A BMX bike is nothing like a mountain bike. A BMX is very small, with a low seat. These bikes are not made for racing or trails, but are used for jumps and stunts in bike parks. You can jump with a mountain bike at certain times, but it is much more difficult to do tricks using them. If you have ever seen those videos of bike stunts, where they roll and jump off stairs and railings, these are the kinds of bikes they use.

BMX bikes have brakes, of course, but they don't have any gears.

Comparing MTB and Hybrid Bikes

Hybrid bikes are in-between a mountain bike and a road bike, and are best for everyday riding. People usually buy these types of bicycles to get to-and-from work or school. These bikes are made to ride comfortably with little effort, but still allow you to ride on trickier paths. That means the tires are wider than a road bike, but not quite as big as a mountain bike.

Comparing MTB and E-Bikes

In short, E-bikes have a battery, and that does a lot of the pedaling work for you. It is basically a cross between a mountain bike and a scooter. The point of these bikes is to allow you to set it so that it gets easier and easier to pedal. The problem is that these bikes are extremely heavy, and you have to charge them before every ride.

For youngsters, e-bikes aren't necessary! These bikes are best for slightly older riders, or riders who have had an injury to their body and can't take the strain of normal pedaling.

Chapter 2:

Getting to Know Your Mountain

Bike

Getting to know your bike for a better ride

By getting familiar with all the parts and pieces of a mountain bike, you can change the bike and all its controls to make your riding even better. By understanding how all the parts work, you can start to look out for certain things that may prevent you from riding at your full potential.

Understanding the Frame

The bike's frame is made to hold all the bike parts together. It is basically the big metal triangle without the wheels, chains, and brakes.

Each type of bike has its own shape, depending on what it will be used for. There are many different types of materials used to make the frame—aluminum, steel, or carbon steel—and each of them has its own benefits.

Aluminum and steel bikes are very hardy and don't crack or break easily. The only problem is that they are a little heavier than carbon steel, for instance. But the frames on mountain bikes are made so that you sit more upright than road bikes, which helps you control them better on trails.

Understanding the Frame Sizes

Mountain bike frames come in a few different sizes, and you can choose your size based on your height. It is important to get the right size, since too big or too small sizes can cause injury, or just a really bad riding experience.

Measure yourself to see what size frame you should get.

- If you are between 4' 10" - 5' 2" (148cm - 158cm) get an **extra-small** frame.
- If you are between 5'3" - 5'6" (159cm - 168cm) get a **small** frame.
- If you are between 5'6" - 5'9" (168cm - 175cm) get a **medium** frame.
- If you are between 5' 11" - 6' 1" (179cm - 185cm) get a **large** frame.
- If you are between 6' 2" - 6' 4" (186cm - 193cm) get an **extra-large** frame.

Understanding the Gears and Brakes

The gears on your bike will completely change the way you ride. By using your gears, you can go faster on flat roads, and be able to climb hills more easily. You can change your gears using the shifters on your handlebars. Later in the book, you will learn exactly how to use these gears for better cycling.

Some bikes have two sets of gears, a small gearset and a bigger one. When there are two groupsets, you will hear that they speak of "a-two-by-twelve" (2X12) or a "two-by-nine (2X9)," for example. What that means is that there are two gear sets, and different speeds for each set. But we talk about this in more detail further on in the book.

When it comes to your brakes, there are two levers on the front of your handlebar which control your brakes. One of your hands will control your front-wheel brake, and your other hand will control your back wheel. This is important because when you learn to do specific skills, knowing which hand controls which brake will help you ride better and keep yourself from falling off.Suppose you aren't sure which hand controls which brake; simply test it. Do this by walking and pushing the bike next to you. Pull one of your levers really hard to stop the bike. You will see and feel which wheel stops dead, and you'll know which lever is connected to which brake. Usually, the back wheel is controlled by the right hand, and the front wheel is controlled by the left hand, but just check in any case.

Understanding the Wheels and Tires

There are a few different types and sizes of tires available when it comes to wheels. But the major thing to know is that you can have a tubular tire and a tubeless tire. Many people will tell you different things, but you should know that tubeless tires have the most benefits. The best of these is that you can change any type of tire and make them tubeless.

This is important for a few reasons. Firstly, tubeless tires ride better and smoother on rough roads. But most importantly, they are a lot easier to fix. With tubeless tires, you have a smaller chance of getting a flat tire while riding, and they are easier to fix if you have a puncture. In fact, if there is a small puncture hole, your tubeless tire fixes itself! Tubeless tires have sealant on the inside which fills your small holes automatically without you even knowing there was a hole.

There are a few to choose from when it comes to tire sizes, and each of them has its own benefits and downsides.

- **26-inch wheels** - This is the most common wheel size. They are light, and you can quickly gain momentum on flat surfaces. But when you compare this to bigger sizes, the 26-inch wheels don't have as much traction or stability.
- **27-inch wheels** - This wheel is great since it is more stable, and slightly smoother than the 26er, but also still easy to handle and flick.
- **29-inch wheel** - these wheels are quickly becoming very popular since they roll really well over rocks and roots. They are best for rough roads, but aren't the first choice for quick flicking and moving.

Pumping Your Tires

An important part of cycling is keeping your tires pumped. These tire pumps are not expensive, especially when you buy them second-hand. It is important to keep your tires at the proper pressure so that you have the best grip and traction. But most importantly, the wrong pressure can be dangerous.

If your tire pressure is too low, you can hurt your tires, and you will need to replace them sooner. If the pressure is very low, you can even damage your actual wheel, which will cost a lot more to replace. But if there is too much air in them, you can crack the outside of the rubber, which also means you will need to replace it.

1. To pump your tires, take off the dust cap (which is the small black cap).
2. With some bikes, there is a small valve underneath the cap, which you also have to loosen. Be very gentle because they can break easily.
3. Now you can put the pump head over the valve and clip it in.
4. Press the pump once, and see what your tire pressure is.
5. The back tire should be between 1.9-2 bars (28-30psi), and the front should be 1.7-1.9 bar (26-28psi).

6. When you are done, make sure you take the pump head off carefully, and tighten the valve and dust cap again.

Understanding the Handlebars

Handlebars are an extremely important part of your bike, since it is how you steer. Even the simplest changes to your handlebars will make a massive difference to how you ride.

Most mountain bike handlebars are long and flat. These handlebars can be shortened if necessary, making your bike much easier to handle. When buying your bike, let them help you measure your arm length and handlebars so that they are your perfect length. You want your handlebars to be quite short, so you don't hit any obstacles on single trails. But you don't want themso short that it is uncomfortable to reach your controls.

Understanding the Seat, Saddle, and Dropper Post

When you ride, you can spend hours on your saddle, so it is really important to find yourself a comfortable saddle with padding. If you are just starting with mountain biking, the best saddles are cushioned. They are best for all the bumps in the roads, and for long times on your seat.

You can start looking at different saddles when you enter competitions or races, or start downhill racing.

Under your saddle, a long, metal pole holds your seat in place as part of your bike frame. This is usually set up at a perfect height for you, and stays like that all the time. But there is a different type of seat post, known as a 'dropper post,' which lets you move your seat all the way down and up while you are on the trails.

If you are serious about mountain bike riding, you should try to get yourself a dropper soon. You can learn how to use a dropper for downhills or tricky roads. By dropping the seat down, it is out of your way, and allows you to move around on your bike more freely. And best of all, you can control the movement of your post with a simple button on your handlebar.

Understanding the Pedals

Your pedals are another part of your bike that will make a massive difference in how you ride. As a rider, you can choose between flats or clipped pedals (also known as cleats). With cleats, your shoes clip into the pedals, so they basically become part of your foot. When it comes to rough roads or climbs, cleats are better for controlling your bike.

Flats are for regular pedals, where you just rest your foot on the pedal. These are the better option for beginners, since you can put your foot down at any time you feel unsteady. You also don't need any special shoes for flat pedals.

Understanding Suspension

If you look at the basic frame of a bike, it is a triangle frame of metal pipes. This is designed so you can sit comfortably with two wheels at the bottom that turn when you pedal.

As the years passed, experts found ways to change the bike so that wasn't so bumpy and hard when you rode down rocky roads. They added something we call a 'suspension,' which almost acts like a spring.

These shocks on the suspension protect the rider from shaking too much on bumps.

Here are the different types of suspensions you can choose from.

Hardtail Bikes

These bikes only have one suspension (shock) above the front wheel. These are slightly more comfortable than traditional bikes with no suspension. They also help with downhills, since the suspension helps with some of the bumps and shakes. And since your bike isn't hitting the obstacles as hard as it would with no suspension, your bike lasts longer with less damage.

Full suspension

Other bikes have suspensions in the front but also at the bottom of your seat near your pedals. These are known as 'dual-suspension' or 'full-suspension' bikes. These are great for really bumpy roads to make your ride more comfortable. The dual-suspension bikes are able to spring over rocky areas without knocking too hard into them, or knocking the saddle too hard into you.

Understanding the Bike Components

There are other parts of the bike that are responsible for getting you from point A to point B. These parts of the bike are not something you're going to work with every day, and are the more technical pieces.But it is great to know and understand these pieces so that you will understand what your bike mechanic is talking about. Or better yet, you can buy a bike that fits exactly what you want, since you understand all the technical terms.

Mountain Bike Crankset

Simply explained, the crankset is right by your pedal, and uses your leg movement to turn the chain, which turns your back wheel. A long piece holds your pedal, which is called a crank-arm. And the little spikes on the crankset are called chainrings, which hold and move the chain.

Not all mountain bikes have the same number of chainrings, which can range from a 26-tooth to a 32-tooth.

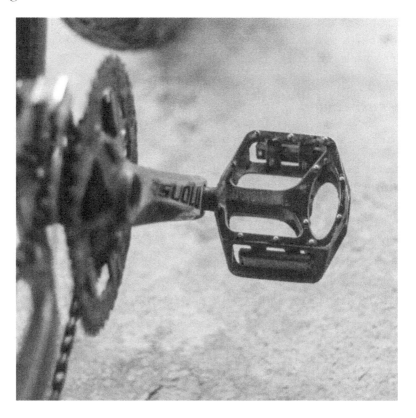

Mountain Bike Cassettes

Your mountain bike cassette is attached to your back wheel, which holds the chain at the back. So your chain is kept on your bike by your crankset and your cassette. Just like the crankset, your cassette has spikes known as sprockets. The number of sprockets you have on your cassette will differ, depending on how many gears you have.

Comparing 1X bikes with 2X Bike

Have you ever heard someone say "a 2-by" or "1-by-9 bike"?

When you hear that kind of bike-talk, you know they are speaking about the number of chainrings the bike has, and then the number of gears available. These gears also determine the speed options you have. So some bikes will just have one set of chainrings on the bike, which we call a one-by (1X). This also means there will only be one lever on your handlebar for changing gears, which is usually on your right-hand side. This is the simplest method for changing gears, and is becoming the most popular type of bike.

On the other hand, a two-by bike (2X) will have two sets of chainrings, meaning there are quite a few gears to move between. These are great for uphill since there is a smoother riding style on an uphill if you have a 2X bike. Some bikes even have a 3X, which makes your pedaling even easier. So a bike with 2X12 has two gear-sets with twelve different speeds. If you have a 1X9 bike, it only has one gearset with nine speeds.

But if you want to learn how to use your gears for better riding, keep reading!

Mountain Bike Chains

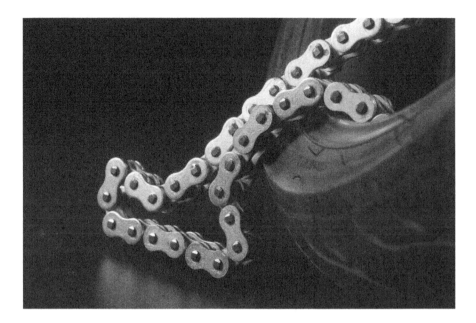

Your mountain bike chain connects your pedal and crankset to your cassette and back wheel, so it is responsible for transferring the power from the pedal to your back-wheel so that your bike can move forward.

There are a few different types of chains, and the one you get will depend on your gears and cassettes. But when you buy a bike, you generally don't have to worry about these pieces. Most bikes come with the correct chain for the right bike.

Understanding Other Accessories

There are a few accessories you can carry with you, which can be helpful on some rides.

- Water bottle holders - most bikes come with one holder, which isn't always enough. So if you are considering far rides, carry a water pack with you.
- Lights - if you are going to be riding at night, it is so important to have a front light (also known as lumens).
- Saddlebags - these are small pouches you can tie to the back of your saddle. This is a must-have when carrying around tools and safety accessories (which we will talk about later).

How to Choose the Right Mountain Bike For You

Now that you know the different bikes you can choose from, and what your bike is made of, you can choose the bike that is made for you.Firstly, think about what you want to be doing on your mountain bike. Do you want to go into enduro, downhill, or general mountain biking? After that, you can start looking at different bike options. Make sure you look at bikes that fit your size and wheel preference.

When you have a few options you like, the best thing you can do is test-ride them. If you buy from a store, they often let you ride the bike first and see if you like it. This is the best thing you can do to see if it is what you are looking for.

As a beginner, you might not be able to feel the differences immediately, but try a few bikes first and see which ones you are most comfortable with.

Chapter 3:

The Mountain Bike Gear You Need

To Get Yourself

The must-have Mountain Bike gear for all beginners

When you start your mountain bike journey, there will be quite a few things you need to buy yourself in the beginning. This gear can sometimes be expensive, but it is important to buy yourself high-quality equipment that will last longer and protect you. Don't get yourself all the cheapest gear in the beginning because you may just have to replace them a few months later. Quality equipment will last a really long time, and keep you safe and injury-free.

Mountain Bike Helmet

The most important gear you can get yourself is a helmet and wear it all the time, no matter how short the ride. Do not underestimate the safety that a helmet can give you. There are a huge variety of helmets, but it is important that you get yourself a helmet from a company that focuses on mountain biking.

A cheap helmet from any sports shop isn't the best idea. You have the option to get a simple helmet that fits on your head or a full-face helmet that also covers your face. These look like motor-cross helmets and are great if you want to do downhill mountain biking.

But when choosing a helmet, there are a few important things to look for that each helmet should have:

The Correct Size

One of the biggest mistakes riders make is buying a helmet that is too big or too small. Make sure you fit on a helmet with the help of someone in the store. Or, measure around your head (just above your eyebrow) and use this chart to find your size.

- If you measure 22.5 - 22 inches, get a small helmet.
- If you measure between 22 - 23.2 inches, get a medium.
- If you measure 23.2 - 23.7 inches, get large.
- If you measure between 23.7 - 25,2, get an extra-large helmet.

Adjustable Straps

Firstly, ensure your helmet has straps that tie around your ears and clip below your chin. But make sure that these straps can be loosened and tightened for a snug fit. You need to adjust your straps to sit quite tightly under your chin. It shouldn't hang loose around your face; otherwise, the helmet is completely useless. When you click closed under your chin, you should be able to open your mouth comfortably but feel it push against your chin when you open up.

Retention System

A retention system is a small knob at the back of the helmet that helps you tighten it around your head. This stops the helmet from moving around while you wear it.

Mountain Bike Shoes

If you are riding with flats, any sports shoe will work fine. But try and get yourself mountain bike shoes because they will give you the best experience. Most of them are designed to grip the pedals so that your feet don't slip off the pedals every time you ride.

Many riders also get cramps in their feet if they wear the wrong shoes because the shoes are too soft, and their toes bend at the front. Many brands specialize in mountain bike shoes, and come in many styles and colors.

If you decide to ride with clips (cleats), you will need to buy clip shoes and pedals specifically. These cleats have a specific design at the bottom, which allows the pedal to clip into the shoe.

Here is a table to compare casual mountain bike shoes and casual riding shoes.

	Mountain Bike Shoes	Casual Riding Shoes
Bottom of the shoe	They have a tread for gripping the pedal	They are smooth
Sole of the shoe	The sole is hard to keep your foot still	The sole is soft so that you can walk in them too
Cleat style	The cleats are built into the bottom of the sole	The cleats are built into the bottom of the sole

Gloves

Gloves are another great addition to your gear since they have a lot of benefits you might not have thought about. Firstly, gloves made for mountain bikers give you extra grip on your handles. Secondly, they help prevent blisters on your hands from holding the handlebars for so long.

Designers have also started making different types of gloves for different uses. Some of them have padding, some are wind-resistant, and others have knuckle protection or are water-resistant. You can get yourself one that fits a lot of different situations.

Cycling Pants

If you're going to be on a mountain bike, you're going to want to get some cycling shorts. If you don't cycle with padded shorts, you will be forever regretful. Sitting on a saddle for hours becomes extremely painful, so you need pants that offer some support and cushioning.

You can get yourself simple cycling pants that you put on like ordinary pants, or you can get yourself a bib that you pull over your shoulders as well. These bibs are great to keep your pants from falling down.

If you don't like the style of the tight mountain biking shorts, you can also get yourself some loose suspension to put over your cycling shorts. These look more like regular pants but let you wear your soft cycling pants underneath.

Cycling Shirts

You can cycle in any type of shirt, but if you want to be more comfortable, try shirts that are specifically made for cycling. Most of them are great for airflow and keeping you cool. Many shirts also come with pockets at the back that work to keep your phone or snacks. So as you become more serious about cycling, you can start getting yourself different cycling shirts.

Biking Sunglasses

You want to wear sunglasses when you're riding, trust me. If you spend a lot of time on the bike, the sun can become very hard to handle, and take your focus off the road. You can get yourself sunglasses specifically for cycling, which help with sun glares, and keeping your eyes focused even when the light changes.

Taking care of your eyes is just as important as taking care of the rest of your body, so don't skip out on some good-quality glasses.

Goggles

Goggles are usually used by hardcore racers who do downhill or enduro racing. With downhill racing, you will usually wear a full-face helmet that protects your head and face while racing. The goggles work better than sunglasses for these races.

If you are racing down a hill you are leaning forward, so you can't really worry about whether your sunglasses are going to fall off, which is why the goggles work best. But if you prefer goggles over sunglasses, you can wear them with any type of mountain biking.

There are a few things to think about when buying goggles to make sure they work for what you need.

Hardiness

With mountain biking goggles, you want something that is not made of metal or glass. If you do fall, those materials can hurt quite a bit if the glasses break. So you are better off wearing the plastic goggles that will be hardy and tough even if you fall.

Color

When choosing goggles, you want clear ones or ones that have a light color. A lens that is too dark will make it difficult for your eyes to adjust when there are shadows or when you ride from lighter to darker areas. Luckily most mountain biking goggles have a lens that still protects your eyes from the sun.

Knee Pads

These pads are optional, but you may want to get yourself a set if you are a beginner. They simply slide over your knees and offer the necessary padding around your knee and part of your shin. This might seem silly in the beginning, but if you do fall on your knee, you can get seriously hurt. And rather safe than sorry, so pad up those knees!

Elbow Pads

Elbow pads are another optional (but recommended) addition to your cycling. They slip on, just like knee pads, and protect the bony part of your elbow. When we fall, we put out our arms to stop the fall (without even realizing we do it). You can seriously hurt yourself if you fall hard on your elbow, so don't take the chance, and keep yourself safe.

Hydration Pack

A hydration pack goes by many different names, like camel pack and water bladder. Whatever you want to call it, they all do the same thing: offer you water.

Your mountain bike will probably have a water bottle holder, but you will need a lot more water if you do long rides. These hydration packs can hold a lot, and best of all, you can add a lot of ice on hot days.

Top Mountain Bike Brands to Choose From

Now that you know what you should look for in a bike, you can choose between the different mountain bike brands that are available. Each brand has its own unique take on bicycles, so here is what you need to know about these brands and what they are like.

Trek

Trek was started in 1975 in Wisconsin and is one of the top mountain biking brands in the world. One of the best things about their brand is that they make bikes of all prices. You will also find other bike brands, like Gary Fisher, Bontrager, and Diamant Bikes, which are all part of Trek's brand.

Giant

Giant is the biggest bike manufacturer in the world and also makes bikes in all price ranges. They have become known for their unique ideas and were the first company to make a large number of carbon frames. If you are looking for a popular brand that has a good reputation for quality bikes, Giant is a good brand to try.

Specialized

Specialized was started in California, where they first started making bike parts. When they started making complete bikes, they focused on making specialized bikes for serious riders. They are one of the biggest carbon steel users, and have started using technology in many of their newest bikes.

Mongoose

Just like Trek, Mongoose was started in Wisconsin in the 1970s, and first focused on making BMX bikes. As their business started to grow, they started making mountain bikes that you can find in many stores. Their biggest focus is on entry-bikes that you can buy anywhere, but they also make specialized mountain bikes you have to buy online.

Chapter 4:

How to Set Up Your Bike

The Correct Bike Set Up For Better Riding

If you want to get the best out of your mountain bike experience, you should set your bike up perfectly. Not all people are the same, so not all bikes are set up the same. But when you understand how you should set up your own bike, you will have the best riding experience.

We suggest that you have a professional help you set up your entire bike, but in the beginning, here are some ways you can set up your own bike yourself.

Saddle Height

Setting your seat and your saddle at the correct height is extremely important. Not only will it help you ride better, but it will prevent any long-term issues. If you pedal and your seat is too high or too low, you can hurt yourself unnecessarily.

Here is what can happen if you don't set your saddle correctly:

- Knee pain - if your knee is straining, you can damage your knee joint with the pushing and pulling of your pedal.
- Hip pain - just like with your knee, with a saddle that is too high, there is too much strain on your hip.
- Lower back pain - if your saddle is too low or high, you will sit too far forward or too straight, which can hurt your lower back.

- Hamstring issues - Your saddle height can hurt the mussels in the back of your legs, and cause constant cramping.

Do you see why it is important to set your seat height correctly?

The best thing would be to get professional help with your bike setup and seat height. But you can check the height yourself by standing next to your bike. If your saddle is at your hip bone, your seat is at the right height.

If it isn't touching your hip bone, you need to set it that way. You can loosen your seat post with an Allen key, and make it higher or lower. You can find an Allen key on your multi-toolkit (which you can read about in chapter 7).

Another way to test your seat height is by sitting on your bike while it is standing still. You can ask someone to hold the bike up while you do this. Put your heel on the pedal and straighten one of your legs completely. Your knee should not be bent at all. If there is a bend, it means your seat is too low.

Once your seat is slightly higher, put the front of your foot on the pedal. Now there should be a very small bend in your knee. This gentle bend when you pedal is just so that your knee never "locks out,' and straightens completely.

Angle of Saddle

Many experts will tell you many different things about how your saddle should be angled. Should it be perfectly straight? Should it be tilted slightly upwards or slightly downwards?

The answer is, it depends on you. For beginners, a perfectly straight saddle is the best angle. When you become more comfortable on the bike, you can test out different angels. Many riders who enjoy uphills say that they like their seat tilted down. Other riders who do downhill racing, like their seat tilted up. So start with your seat on a neutral level, and first just get the hang of the basics.

Bar Height

The height of your handlebar is important because it allows your elbows to be at the right angle all the time. Like with your knees and hips, it is important that your elbows are at the correct angle to prevent injury. But you will have to ask a professional to help see where your handlebar should be, since they measure all parts of your body to see what your individual height should be.

With handlebars, however, you can set them slightly higher or lower depending on what kind of riding you want to do. Here is what we mean:

- **Lower handlebars:** Setting your bar lower means you have more weight in the front of your wheel, which is excellent for quick cornering. But this isn't a great position if you are trying to climb steep hills.
- **Higher handlebars:** These are great for more control on steep hills, and it is overall a more comfortable position.

So unless you will be focusing specifically on tight corners and downhills, ask the professionals to keep your handlebar fairly high.

Brake Levers

All of the controls on your bike (like your brakes, gears, and dropper control) can be set up on the handlebar to fit you best. The most important thing is that you can rest at least one finger on your brakes *at all times.* You have to get used to riding with your fingers on the brakes, so that you can brake if anything happens. So the angle of your brakes needs to be comfortable for your wrists.

When you hold your handlebars and straighten your arms, you should be able to stick out your pointer finger and grab the edge of the brake lever (where it curves). You don't want to have to twist your wrists to reach your levers.

Other Controls

Other than your brake levers, you have your dropper post, gears, and shock lockout button.

You can decide what you are most comfortable with when it comes to each control. But the most common set-up is to put your dropper post control on your right handlebar close to your thumb at the bottom of the bar.

Depending on how many gears you have, you will either have one or two controls. These are most commonly put close to your thumb too, but at the top of your handlebars.

If you have a bike with full suspension, you can lock out your shocks by using a button on your handlebar. This is not something you use as often as your gears or brakes, so it is usually set up on the left handlebar at the top.

So if you lock your shocks, it means your bike doesn't bounce around and roll over rocks as easily. You will generally only lock your shocks when you are going uphill, so that you have more traction.

You can leave your shocks in the middle when you are just doing everyday riding, so that there is a good combination between traction but also rolling over bumpy parts.

You will completely unlock your shocks when you are going downhill, so that your bike is able to easily roll over the rocky parts without shaking you too much.

Chapter 5:

The Five Things to Never Forget

When Riding

The 5 Basic MTB Rules to Get Started

Getting On-and-Off

You might think getting on and off is the easiest part about riding, right? Well, you will be surprised how many adults still don't know how to get on and off a bike correctly.

"Why does it matter," you may ask. It matters because if you ever do decide to do mountain biking races, and something happens on the trail that forces you to stop and get off, you want to do it quickly. If you are in a race, everything needs to happen at super speed, and getting on and off can affect your time.

So if you want to make sure you get this right, here is what you should do:

Getting On

1. If you are riding with flats, it is much easier to get on and off your bike.

2. Stand on the left side of your bike and hold your handlebars. It is best to get on from the left side so that you don't get oil on you (from the chain).
3. Lean forward toward your handlebars and swing your right leg over the saddle.
4. Now you will be standing over the bike with the bike in between your legs.
5. When you want to start moving the bike, use your foot to pull the right pedal up. This is so that you can 'push'" yourself away and get some momentum.
6. Make sure you look ahead to where you want to steer. Don't look down at your feet.
7. When the pedal is slightly higher, put your right foot on the pedal, and use your left foot to push yourself away from the ground.
8. When you pedal for the first time, use the momentum to stand up straight, and sit on the seat.

It may seem like many steps to follow just to get on, but it is really easy. All you have to do is try it a few times, and you'll do great!

Getting Off

Getting off is just as important as getting on. You want to get off as safely and smoothly as you can.

1. If you see the area you want to stop at, start braking slowly with both hands.
2. As your bike starts to come to a stop, stand up on your pedals and push your hips forward.
3. Now you can take your right leg off the pedal and slowly put it down on the ground. You will then be in the same position that you started.

4. From this position, you can get back onto your seat quickly and smoothly.
5. This also takes a lot of practice because you have to get used to standing, stopping, and being comfortable with how slow your bike can go without falling over.

Chin Up

As a mountain biker, the most important thing you need to do whenever you are cycling, wherever you are cycling, is keep your chin up and your eyes ahead.

When you first start riding your bike, you are going to want to look right in front of you. You still feel shaky and scared on your bike, and that's normal. But no matter where you are, you have to practice looking out ahead in front of you to see what else is 'coming your way.'

Mountain bike trails are filled with surprises—jumps, turns, hills, rocks, and roots. You have to keep your chin up and eyes ahead so you can prepare yourself if you need to turn quickly, or go over an obstacle.

You should regularly look at where you are going right then, and then just look up for a few seconds to see what's ahead. Practice scanning the area constantly.

Keep Your Eyes on the Road You Want to Go

One of the biggest mistakes that new riders make is that they look at the obstacles that they are scared of.

Don't ever look at anything else except the road you want your bike to go on.

When you start riding, you will notice that you and your bike become one. So, where you look is where your bike will go. If there are rocks that you don't want to ride over, *don't* look at them. If you are riding over a bridge, *don't* look at the sides of the bridge. Just look at the single path you want to keep your bike on.

Of course, this is a lot easier said than done. It is sometimes a habit to look at the things that we are scared of on a trail. But you have to practice keeping your eyes ahead and keeping your eyes on the road you want the bike to stay on.

Your Feet Positioning

So now that you know how to get on your bike and how to keep yourself in a straight line while riding, there are a few other things that will make it easier for you to ride.

One of the key things is your feet positioning on the pedal. The way your feet sit on the pedal will make a big difference in the way you ride.

Firstly, you have to put the ball of your foot on the pedal. You can't put the pedal in the middle of your foot. Using the ball of your foot (which is the hard part below your toes) gives you more stability and pedaling power.

If you use cleats, your foot automatically slips into these clips, and the ball of your foot will be on the pedal. But if you are wearing flats, you have to practice this position. Sometimes your foot will move, or sometimes you won't get your foot on precisely the right spot. But when you get on your bike, you just have to keep practicing placing your foot on the right spot so it becomes a habit.

Point Your Toes Up and Press Your Heels Down

Part of having your foot in the correct position is how you angle it. Throughout your time on your bike, you need to push your heels down and point your toes toward the sky.

Pushing your heels down toward the ground with your toes pointing up is important for controlling your movements. It also makes sure your body is in the correct position on the bike, and your weight is equally distributed.

If you are riding uphill, keep your heels down. If you are on a flat road, also keep your heel down. But one of the most important places to keep your heels down is on a downhill.

Later in the book, we discuss some tips and tricks for better control on downhills.

Keep Pedaling

If you've ever watched *Finding Nemo*, you will remember one of the scenes where Dorey reminds Marlin to *just keep swimming*.

Remember that every time you cycle. *Just keep pedaling.*

If you find yourself struggling uphill, do NOT stop pedaling. The moment you lose momentum, you have to work much harder going up the hill.

If you find yourself at an obstacle or a turn that looks difficult, don't brake completely. It is normal to be afraid of the turns and the obstacles at first. Everyone has that fear in the beginning. But the worst thing you can do is brake when you feel afraid. When you are on a mountain bike, the momentum and the movement of the bike are what will keep you on the bike.The moment the bike's wheels stop turning is when the biker loses stability and falls over. So if you are afraid, it is okay to slow down a little bit, but don't ever stop dead. Keep pedaling and trust yourself. It is when most people hesitate that they fall.

Take it slow, keep your eye on the path you want to go, and just keep the momentum.

Your Arms and Core

If you want to keep yourself strong and stable on a bike, you need to keep your arms and stomach muscles strong. Throughout the ride, try and keep your stomach muscles tight, which is surprisingly helpful for keeping your bike stable.

If you want to become a professional cyclist, it is important to do exercises that will help keep your stomach muscles strong since it plays such a big role in your riding abilities. We have some great exercises you can do to strengthen these muscles in chapter 8.

When it comes to your arms, there are different positions to put your arms in, which will help improve your riding. So how you keep your arms when you ride uphill will be different from how they will be when you ride downhill.

Here's how you should keep your arms for the best riding experience.

Uphills

Many riders think they should stand off their seat when they're riding up a hill. This does help a little, but puts a lot of stress on your legs.

When you're standing out of the saddle, you are using *only* your leg power to move your bike. And if it is a challenging hill, you're going to tire yourself out extremely quickly.

The best thing to do to get up a hill is to use your entire body so that it isn't just your legs that are responsible for getting yourself up. When you are riding up a hill, you should tuck your elbows in, and press them against your ribs. This will help you tug on your handlebars and use your arms, core, and legs to move the bike.

In the next chapter, there is more detail about riding up a hill, but this is the most important part to remember about your arm positioning.

Downhills

When you ride downhills, you will position your whole body differently. Going downhill, you need to move your weight the right way to prevent yourself from falling over the handlebars. So on a downhill, it is important to stand off your saddle and push your heels down.

Your arms should also be pushed outward, which helps better control your steering. So think of pushing your elbows out all the way out so that they are parallel with your handlebars. You will also drop your chest towards the handlebar, which will automatically push your elbows out, but we will discuss that later on.

For now, just remember that your elbows are out when you go downhill, but your elbows are in when you're going up. In both cases, uphill and downhill, you need to remember to keep one finger on either break. Many riders clench the handlebars tightly since going uphill or downhill can be quite scary. But try not to grip the handlebars too tightly; it can cause your hands to cramp or tire out your forearms.

Chapter 6:

The Best MTB Skills To Practice

The mountain biking skills you'll need for every ride.

No matter which mountain bike you've decided to ride, or what type of trail you've decided to go on, there are some skills you will need to learn. These skills will take you from being a beginner to becoming a pro.

There are a few ways you can change your gears, or go around corners, but if you practice the skills we have in this chapter you will become a really great cyclist. It's all about understanding the bike, and how your body works with the bike.

If you want to know how some riders become world champions, all you have to do is take a look at their skills and techniques. You will see that they just have some small techniques in their body-and-bike movement, making them better than all their competitors.

Balance

Balance is the number one skill that you have to practice if you want to become a better rider. Without balance, how are you going to stay on your bike? Having great balance makes you more comfortable, which is important for riding any type of bike.

You can practice a few things that will help you keep your balance the next time you try out some trails.

Getting Out of Your Saddle

When you're riding downhill, you're going to want to stand up out of your saddle so that you're in better control of your bike. So, if you're not used to standing up on your pedals while you ride, you will want to practice this first.

It feels scary at first. You have a seat for a reason, right? But when you start practicing standing, you will see that it is really the best way to ride specific trails.

So, when you get started, just practice riding on flat ground. You can do a few different things to get you comfortable. You should see how it feels to pedal while you're standing. You can also pedal and get yourself some momentum, and then practice standing while you're not pedaling. Try standing while you go uphill to see how it feels, and also try standing while going down a small hill. Just get comfortable with the idea that you don't have to be glued to your saddle all the time.

Separating Yourself From the Bike

Hang on! Didn't we just talk about how you and your bike become one? So why do you need to separate yourself from the bike?

One of the things you will learn later on in your mountain bike journey is body-and-bike separation. You have to learn to be comfortable with moving your bike in crazy ways underneath you, without feeling that you have to hold on to your bike for dear life. Once you've practiced standing on your pedals, this will be easier to try.

When you start riding downhill, especially when you are comfortable with riding fast, you need to move your bike a lot. With some bumpy trails, you will see how the experts stand on their bikes and move their hips completely to the side, or completely to the back. Some riders are so comfortable that they can hold onto their handlebars and sit on their back wheel at the same time!

So when you practice separating yourself from the bike, just ride in a small area on a flat road. A parking lot or empty field will work great.

Just ride slowly, and move your body all around. Really, *just move*. Move your hips, move your arms, lean forward, and lean back. Get used to the idea that you can move your body all around the bike, and it feels completely normal and comfortable.

You will see many pro-riders do this, so have a look at some videos, and you'll see what we mean. When going around corners, they'll push their bike all the way to the right-hand side, and completely hang off the left-hand side. It looks crazy, and it seems dangerous, but it is doable! And once you get comfortable with the idea that your bike will still go where you want it to, even if you aren't sitting on the saddle, nothing can stop you!

Don't rush through, though. Getting your balance and feeling comfortable separating yourself from the bike takes time and lots of practice. It might take you a few weeks or even months, and that's okay. Just keep practicing, and don't give up.

Riding As Slow as Possible

One of our most important lessons is always to keep pedaling, and to keep your momentum, because that's how you stay on the bike. But sometimes you might have a slow rider in front of you, and you need to keep your balance for a short while without moving much. What also happens is that on really tight corners, you can't ride really fast, and need to move extremely slowly to get around that corner. It's these moments that you are going to wish you had better balance, so that your bike doesn't fall to the side while you're trying to ride slowly, and so that you can practice staying upright.

A great way to practice this balancing skill is to pedal as slowly as you possibly can. You can do this anywhere, since it doesn't take a lot of space.

Your bike can easily stay upright when you're moving quickly. That's how bikes were designed. But once your bike stands still, it naturally falls over. So your task is to pedal *extremely slowly* to challenge your body to keep the bike upright. You will see that this task will work your core muscles—which is another reason you should consider also doing ab-workouts.

If you practice this a few times a week, you will have a lot more stability and balance on the bike. And if you ever find yourself on a trail where you need to move slowly for whatever reason, you're not going just to fall off. If you're comfortable with keeping your bike upright, even when it is hardly moving, you're one step closer to pro-riding.

Standing Still

A bike is bound to fall over when it stands still, right? But there is actually a trick to keeping your bike upright, even when it isn't moving. It's a skill called a *Track-stand,* which is not easy to do, but you should try anyway.

So if you try this at first, and you don't get it right, don't worry. There are many, *many* professional riders who can't do a trackstand. It takes a lot of practice and a lot of frustration, but you're going to thank yourself for it!

Step 1: To try this skill, slow down your bike as much as possible. Stand up out of your saddle, and push your heels down. While you hold your handlebar, try not to put your weight on your arms. Instead, put most of your weight on your feet and your pedals.

Step 2: If you keep your wheel straight, the bike will fall over. As we said, it's how bikes are designed. So you're going to cheat the design. You're going to turn your wheel toward the foot that you pushed to the front when you stopped the bike. That is your leading foot, and you want your wheel to turn towards the leading foot.Some people lead with their left and others with their right, so just find which foot you're most comfortable with having in the front.

Step 3: Without some sort of movement, you will lose your balance and fall over. The trick with a track-stand is to keep moving the bike slightly underneath you. You're going to keep moving your feet back and forth, so your bike rolls to the front a little, and then rolls to the back. So you won't be dead still; uou're going to be moving the bike back and forth a few inches.

Tip: Don't look at your feet when you do this. It is natural to want to do soto see if you're doing it right. But it is important to look ahead and keep yourself on the bike.

Your feet never do a complete turn on the pedals. You are basically just tapping one foot, then the other.

Just like with slow riding, you can practice a track-stand anywhere. Try to get a completely flat road, so you don't have anything that will cause you to fall. A parking lot or driveway is a perfect area.

Keep practicing! Not many cyclists can stay on a bike if it isn't moving. So this will not only be a great skill to have when you are on a trail, but it's a great trick to show your friends.

Gear Changing

Changing your gears, which we also call shifting, is a skill that surprisingly few people have. Your gears are there to help you ride easier on the uphills, and help your bike with stability on the rockier parts.

Everyone can shift their gears up or down with just a click on their handlebars. But not everyone knows the little techniques and skills you can learn to use the gears for excellent riding. There are certain ways you can use your gears that will help you more than you know. Just understanding what your gears do will mean that you can get up a hill that might have been impossible in the past. Trust me; I have firsthand experience with this.

But in any situation when you are shifting gear, don't change them if you are not going to pedal. When you press the gear-shifter, your legs have to be moving so that the chain goes onto the correct gear. If you keep changing gear without pedaling, there is a big chance that your chain will fall off, which will force you to get off and fix it.

So, the golden rule is, don't shift gears unless you're pedaling.

So, what are you meant to do with the gears on your ride?

Riding Flat Roads (1X-Bike)

If you have a 1X bike, it means you only have one cassette, and you only have one lever on your handlebar to change gears. Here, when riding a flat road or a trail, you have to start finding your middle gear. This is the gear that you can pedal in comfortably, without much effort. But it cannot be a gear that is too easy, because if you need to speed up quickly, an easy gear will make you spin on one spot. This means your tire moves, but you're not going anywhere.

So when you see a trail or flat road coming up, put yourself in middle gear, and just keep pedaling. There will probably be a few areas where you don't have to pedal, and you can just glide through the trails. Those parts of the trail are the perfect areas to start practicing your other techniques, like standing.

Riding Flat Roads (2X-Bike)

If you have a 2x bike, which means there are two chainrings and two levers on your handlebar, you will just have one extra thing to think about.

With most bikes, the big cassette's lever is on your right handlebar with most bikes, even if you have a 1X. But with a 2X, you will also have the lever on the left handlebar, which will shift your other set of gears.

So, when you ride on a flat road, you can find a middle gear with your right lever, just like with a 1X bike. The gear makes it easy to pedal on any surface without much effort. But with the left hand lever, you want to change the gear so that you're on the hardest gear. Usually, you do that by pressing the black lever all the way back with your thumb.

You won't feel like you are working harder if you make this gear difficult this way. You will actually see that your bike rides much smoother, and you don't have to pedal as hard to get your bike to move quickly.

You can keep your bike on this gear on your left all the time when you ride on flat surfaces or downhills. It is a safe gear to stay in to help you glide smoothly. It also makes it easier to think only about the right hand gears. These are the ones you will change quite often.

Uphill Riding (1X-Bike)

When you are riding uphill, there are certain things you can do with your gears to make it easier to get up certain steep parts.

If you have a 1X bike, it is quite simple to get to the top of the hill.

Firstly, start off on a gear that is a medium-difficulty level for you. This means that you still have to use a lot of leg power to pedal, but it doesn't feel like you can't pedal at all. Remember that you need to tuck your elbows in, keep your core strong, and *keep pedaling*.

If it is a difficult uphill, you will feel that your energy is dropping, and your legs are starting to burn. But you cannot stop pedaling, or you will fall over! So, if you do start getting tired, press your gears and shift into an easier gear. Your legs won't have to push as hard to get up the hill, and your legs will start to pedal a little faster.

Be careful not to put yourself into easier gear too soon, though. You don't want an easy gear that makes your legs move really quickly. Because when you are going up a hill and pedaling quickly, your legs won't hurt as much. However, you are using a lot of energy and you are doing a lot of cardio, so you will definitely get tired more quickly.

So, better start on a gear that is slightly more difficult, and slowly make it easier and easier for yourself.

Each time you feel your energy dropping, shift down one gear, then another, until you are on the easiest gear. When you can't gear down anymore, *just keep pedaling* and don't stop! You are going to become tired, and your legs are going to hurt. But if you want to become a better mountain bike rider, you have to learn how to keep pedaling and moving, even when it gets hard!

And don't start shifting down with your gears until you absolutely need to. Eventually you're going to want to go on to your easiest gear, and when you choose to do that, make sure it's only when you get close to the end of the hill. Otherwise, you're going to burn yourself out, and you'll want to get off and walk it!

Uphill Riding (2X-Bike)

When it comes to a 2X-bike, you will probably get up a hill easier than someone with a 1X-bike. All your extra gears mean you can make it easier and easier for yourself all the way to the top.

When you start with an uphill, you can start in a slightly harder right-hand gear. Don't start in middle gear. Starting on a harder right-hand gear means, though, that you have to put some effort into your pedaling for the first few seconds. This is important, because when you change your left-hand gear, you will immediately feel a big difference.

When things start getting difficult up the hill, click your left-hand gear once. There will be an immediate change in your effort, and you will feel your pedaling power at a medium difficulty level.

Now, just as with a 1X bike, you will slowly change your right-hand gear, one gear at a time. As you start feeling tired, gear down one and keep pushing, until you have to gear down again.

If you are on a really difficult hill, you will see that your left-hand and right-hand gears are on their easiest. There will be no more clicks to make it easier, and that's when you just have to keep pedaling. Your legs are going to move really quickly, but you won't feel your leg muscles hurt as much.

When you ride like this, with both gears on their easiest, you are in your 'granny gear.' It is a really fun name that cyclists call this easy gear on an uphill. If you struggle uphill, you will just have to *granny the hill*!

Downhill Riding

When you ride downhill, you won't be shifting your gears at all. There is a good chance that you will probably just be *free-riding*, which means you won't be pedaling. The momentum of the bike going down a hill is enough. In that case, you won't need to change your gears either. All you need to be worried about is positioning your body correctly, keeping your chin up, and using your body to move your bike over the obstacles.

This is also a good instance of when your chain can fall off your bike. When you're going downhill, you won't be pedaling, so if you keep changing your gears, the chain might jump off. The one thing to remember is that when you are done with your downhill, and you want to sit down and start pedaling again, you are going to have to quickly gear into a harder gear.

If you were going down the hill quickly, you had a lot of momentum and speed. So, if you are in an easy gear and you start pedaling, your legs are going to spin and you're not going to be able to really get to pedal. Just shift into a harder gear so that you have some power, and your bike can get some grip on the ground.

Uphills

We've shown you some tricks throughout the book for getting up a hill correctly. Now, though, we're going to put all those pieces together for you here, so that you know exactly what to do on an uphill.

Let's say you've been riding on a trail (in your middle gear, of course), and you look ahead to see an uphill. You can quickly run through your uphill checklist in your head to make sure you can ride up there like a pro.

If you have a 1X, you're going to stay in your middle gear for a while. When you see the uphill coming, try to pedal quicker towards the hill so you have some momentum up the first part of the hill. If you have a 2X bike, click your right-hand gear two or three times to make it hard to pedal. This is just so that you can make your left-hand gear very easy, but without losing your momentum. If your bike has suspension, you will have that lever on your handlebar which locks your shocks, remember? Now is the perfect time to lock your shocks, so that your wheel doesn't bounce around anymore, because locking your shocks means your tire pushes down harder on the ground, making it a little easier to pedal.

Now, whatever bike you're riding, you will have to remember your biking rules. Pull your elbows against your ribs; push your chest down a little and stay sitting on the saddle; push your heels down; and keep your chin up and keep pedaling. Remember that the reason you're pulling your elbows against your ribs while sitting down is so that you can use your arms and stomach muscles to get you up the hill. Don't stand and try to pedal up, because you are just tiring yourself quickly. The trick is to pull on your handlebars. Don't pull up towards the sky, but pull down toward your hips. With every pedal, give your handlebar a pull toward your hips, and take deep breaths. You've got this!

As your legs get tired, click your right-hand gear. Try to stay on the harder gears for as long as possible, and keep tugging. Once your energy is almost completely done, put your bike in the granny gear, but don't stop pedaling!

If you're riding up a really steep hill, all this is going to be difficult, especially if it is your first time, or if you're not used to hills. Don't get frustrated with yourself if you struggle. Everyone struggles at the beginning, and not everyone gets to the top the first time. It takes practice, and it's okay to be a beginner.

The most important thing is that you're trying and you're not giving up. If you get too tired, and feel that you have to get off while going uphill, *that's okay!* We all do it sometimes. Even if you walk up most of the hill, the important thing is that you tried.

The more you practice riding up the hill, the stronger your legs will get, and the more you will get used to handling the gears, breathing, pulling, and pedaling. And the day that you get all the way to the top of the hill without getting off, is the day you will be unbelievably proud of yourself. The feeling of riding to the top of a hill by yourself is amazing. It is what mountain biking is all about—and you will get there too. Just keep trying, keep pedaling, and keep your chin up!

Downhill

Like we said earlier, riding downhill will be completely different than uphill.

With an uphill, your elbows are in, and you're sitting down. With downhills, you have to be standing with your elbows pointing out.

Let's imagine you're on the trail again. You're pedaling, your heels are down, and your chin is up. When you look ahead to see what happens to the trail, you see that there is a long downhill on the trail. Just like with an uphill, you can prepare yourself in time, so that you ride down it with no problems.

First, stand up in your saddle. Push your heels down and point your elbows out as far as you can. Lean with your chest down toward the handlebar, and make sure you stick your bum over your saddle. You want your back to be flat and equal so that you are not leaning over your handlebars. If you don't stick your bum out, you might be too forward past your handlebars, which is usually how someone falls on a downhill. You can also unlock your shock, so that your wheel bounces a little on the obstacles.

So, you're going down the hill with your heels down, chin up, bum out and chest down. This is the best position to be to ride down a tricky trail, because you are very stable on the bike. Even if the road is rocky, staying like this will let you ride over the trail easily without losing your balance.

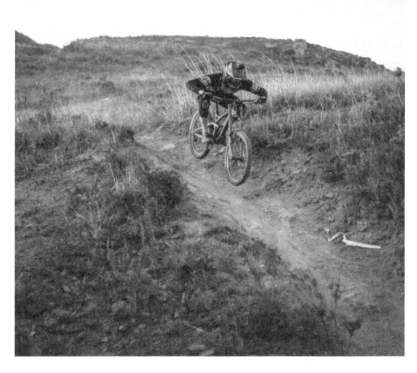

Now, all you have to do is roll over the obstacles while keeping your bike steady. You don't have to pedal, since your bike automatically moves downhill. So stay steady, and move your bike over the rocky sections. If you start going too fast, you can brake a little by using both levers. But when you brake, you have to touch your brake levers very softly. If you pull your brakes hard, your wheels will slide, and you could fall. No matter what part of the trail you're on, always brake very softly, using both your left and right hands. If you only brake the front wheel, sometimes the back wheel will lift and buck you off your bike like a horse!

So, always remember to brake softly, using both hands. And just keep your position all the way down as you roll over the rocks, roots, and stumps.

Sometimes you will see that when pro-riders go downhill, they push themselves all the way to the back, with their bum hanging off the back of their saddle. It looks cool and they ride down the trails really quickly. But that is *not* the best way to ride downhill. By riding like that, you are putting too much weight on the back of the bike, so it will be really easy for the front wheel to lift, and make you fall backward. The position we are teaching you will help you keep all the weight equal on all the parts of the bike, so that the weight is spread out equally, making it easy for your bike to naturally ride down the hill without any reason to fall.

Corners

Corners, corners, corners. It is the part of mountain biking that has most riders fed-up and ready to give up. One of the most difficult parts of mountain biking is going around a sharp corner quickly and safely.

If you want to get better at riding, you have to practice riding the corners. Once you get the hang of it, you're not going to believe how comfortable you'll feel on the trails!

One Elbow in

The most important thing you need to remember when riding any corner is the idea of pulling in your elbows, and pulling yourself toward the handlebars. So if you are turning a corner to your left-hand side, pull your LEFT elbow toward your hip.

If you're going to try and turn your bike with straight arms using your handlebar, it isn't going to go where you want it. There is really no control on turns with your handlebars. Turning your bike where you want it to go means turning your shoulders, hips, and elbows.

So, when practicing going around a corner, pull your elbow against your hip and keep pedaling! You will start to see how comfortable you get, and how much more control you have.

One Knee Out

Once you get the hang of this, you can start adding more techniques. The next step would be to turn your knee out, and point it toward the direction you are going.

So if you're turning a left corner, pull in your left elbow and point your left knee at the corner. Again, there is not a lot of control in your handlebars. Your bike will go to the places you move your elbows, hips, and shoulders. And by pointing your knee toward the corner, you're moving your hips in that direction.

Turning your knee out will take a lot of practice. It takes time to get used to your knee not facing forward. But when you understand how much your bike will be in your control when you're not using your handlebars, you will see a big improvement in your riding.

Straighten the Rest

Alright, so you're turning a left corner. You're tucking your left elbow toward your knee, and you're pointing your left knee toward the left corner. You've got the two most important things going. You should already see a big improvement in the way you're taking corners.

And if you've been doing some balance practices, you should be able to take a corner at a nice and easy speed, without falling over.

Once you get the hang of your knee and elbow, there is one more element to this: your other arm and leg. What happens to your right knee and right elbow if you're turning left?

You straighten them.

Use your right hand to push against the handlebar. And straighten your right leg completely. If you turn to the left-hand side and your left leg is straight, you're going to hit the ground with your pedal. This is known as a pedal-strike.A pedal stroke is the worst way to fall off your bike because it's a silly thing to happen.

So, whenever you're turning to the left, don't straighten your left leg! If you're turning to the right, make sure your right knee is bent. You never want your pedal to be close to the ground around the corner you're turning.

In the beginning, all this will feel like a lot to remember. But just like all other skills, the more you practice, the more natural it will feel after a while.

So, remember: if you're turning right, you will straighten the left side of your body. And the same goes for the other side.

Chin Up

Again, don't forget one of the most important rules of riding: Keep your chin up!

Don't try and check if your elbow is bending correctly, or see if your knee is pointing out enough. Trust yourself and see how it *feels*. But don't try to look at your body, because it will make you lose your balance.

Instead, look at where you want to go, and your bike will take you there.

Berms

When you get comfortable with turning corners, you will be able to start trying out berms.

A berm is basically a corner that has a bit of a hill on the outside of the corner. Sometimes they turn the trail completely on its side. Some trails have berms as high as a wall next to you, and other berms are just small sandbanks.

But no matter what type of berm you are riding, there are some tips and tricks that will help you get comfortable with them, and ride like a pro.

When trying to ride a berm quickly, you have to remember the basic rules of riding.

1. Keep your chin up and look at where you want to go.

2. Tuck in your elbow towards the corner that you're turning.

3. Try pointing your knee toward the corner you are turning.

4. Keep looking ahead so you have an idea of what is going to happen on the trail, especially after the berm.

But when you try doing berms, there are a few other things you have to do that will help you ride better.

First, before you get to the berm, slow down your bike. Then, choose your riding line. That sounds odd to beginners, but it will make sense in a second.

When you ride a berm, the trick is to ride up high onto the berm, and then come out quite low. As you ride toward the berm, draw a line with your eyes, choose where you are going to ride in high, and go out low.

If you look at the picture below, this is the type of line this rider would have chosen for himself. This is the line he drew with his eyes. He rode up high, and will come down low. Notice how he is looking at the 'low' area. He is looking where he wants his bike to go.

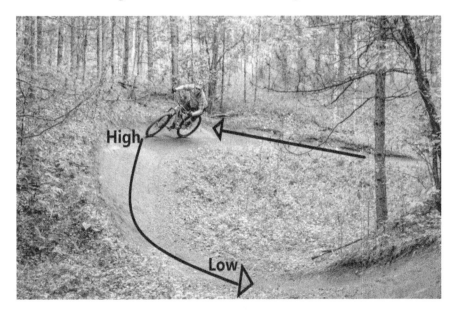

The reason you ride in high is so that you can use the small downhill to get some momentum, and go quickly. This is very useful for races.

You can ride in low and go out low, but you won't have as much speed, and you might need to pedal on the corner. Just be careful not to go in too high and go off the side.

This high-in low-out method is the perfect way to ride a berm. It will take some practice and take some confidence. After all, riding your bike on its side can be scary if you are a beginner, and even if you have been riding for years.

So as you come towards a berm, this is the type of line you should draw for yourself, so that you can look at where you want to go. Where your eyes go, your bike will follow.

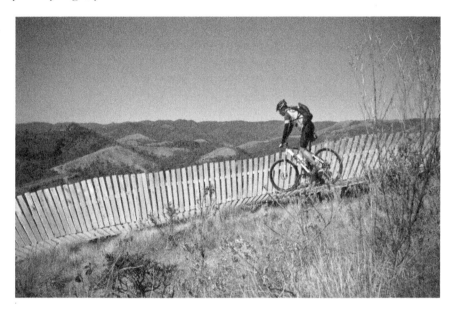

Switchbacks

A switchback is just another word we use for a certain corner of the trail. Switchbacks can be very difficult to do if you don't practice them. Many riders who have been on a bike for years still can't do a switchback.

There is a trick to a switchback that not everyone knows, which is why so many riders still struggle. If you want to learn how to do switchbacks, try these methods and practice them over and over again, until you can do it. Once you get it right the first few times, all the other switchbacks will be a breeze.

What is a Switchback?

A switchback is just a really tight corner on a single track. But you know how to do corners now, don't you? So this will be a breeze!

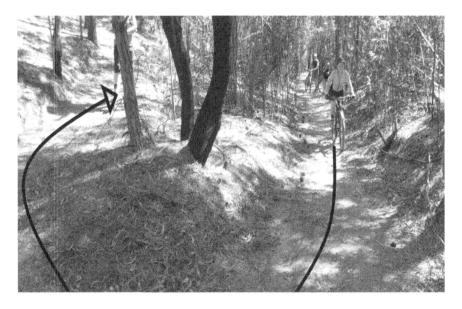

The difference with these corners is that you can't go around them quickly, and will need to go super-slow and use all the techniques you've learned to get it right.

If you are going to be riding a trail up a mountain, you will definitely experience a few switchbacks. It is impossible to build a road straight up a mountain, so they have to make some switchbacks for you to get up. Now you just have to practice, and become a switchback master.

Sometimes a switchback goes up slightly, and other times there are downhill switchbacks. How you ride up a switchback will be slightly different than a downhill. But no matter what your switchback looks like, there are a few things to remember every time.

1. Brake before you get there.

If you were keeping your chin up during your ride, you would have seen that there is a corner or a switchback ahead, which helps you prepare yourself for it. It is important to do most of the braking before you get to the switchback, and not while you are turning on it.

2. Draw your line

When you reach the switchback, you should draw a line for yourself, just like you do with any other corner. Remember that you want to try to go up quite high, and then go out low. You want to go around the switchback as wide as you can to give yourself some room.

3. Tuck your elbow and point your knee

Remember those turning skills you were trying on a corner? Since a switchback is just another corner, you can use those skills here too. Tuck your elbow toward your hip, and point your knee toward the corner. If you are going really, really slowly, it will be more difficult to point your knee. But try and turn it as much as is comfortable.

4. Look at your exit point

When you are riding a switchback, it is natural to want to look down at the road because of how tight the corner is. This is the mistake that most riders make on a switchback, which is why so many can't do it. Keeping your chin up has never been more important than on a switchback. You shouldn't look down *ever*.

Where you look when going around a switchback will be the difference between making it and not making it. So keep your chin up all the way toward the turn. And the moment you start turning, look at where you want to exit the switchback. You have to look at where you want your bike to go, remember? So make sure you do that the entire time you go around the corner.

First look ahead, until you start turning, and then immediately look at your exit. Let's look at the switchback again, and point out exactly where you should look ahead, and where your eyes should be for your exit.

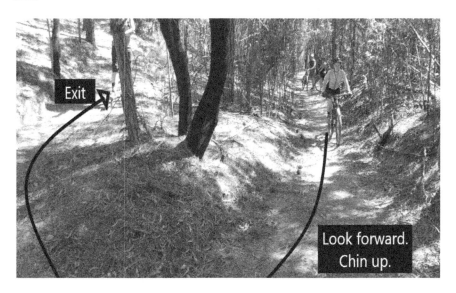

Braking

Braking is supposed to be easy, right? When you're going too fast, you are supposed to brake. But it's not always that simple. Sometimes, if you want to have the best ride, you have to brake at more specific times.

You've seen now that when you want to go around a corner, berm, or switchback, you brake *before* you turn the corner. The reason you brake before the corners, and not at the corners is so that you can focus on your skills, and not need to focus on slowing down too. Also, you need your tire to connect perfectly with the ground on the corner to keep yourself upright. Traction is at its best when your bike is moving, which is why you should brake before the corner.

You also know now that when you go downhill, you have to brake gently and slowly. The same thing applies to traction. Your bike has the best traction when it is moving, so try to keep your bike rolling down the hill, even if it is extremely slow. But you don't want to keep braking all the way down, because that makes the bike lose traction.

So what are the other ways you can brake for a better ride?

Brake With One Finger

No matter what type of mountain bike you're riding, or what trail you are on, it is important to keep one finger on your brakes *all the time.* Remember that if anything happens on the trail, you need to be able to stop in time. And by having your fingers on the brakes, you can stop in time.

The best is just to have one finger on each brake. Brake slowly and softly so that you don't throw yourself off the bike. But if you ride with three or four fingers on the brake, you might pull too hard and brake too suddenly. Also, if you have too many fingers on the brakes, you have less power on the handlebars, making it difficult to control your bike on the trails.

So, one finger is enough. It is up to you if you want to use your middle fingers or your pointer fingers. Try each one and see which one is more comfortable for you.

Brake Before an Obstacle

The turns and berms are also obstacles, and you have to brake before them. But you should brake before you get to any obstacle. If there are any stumps, logs, roots, or rocks in your path, brake before you get to them. Then, roll over them gently. Speed and momentum will keep you on your bike, so if you brake while you are going over the obstacles, you might lose your balance.

So, it is better to brake before the obstacle and not brake while going over it.

Manuals (Front Wheel Lifts)

With a manual, you quickly lift your front wheel to get your bike onto some obstacles that are too high to ride over. If you have ever tried to get onto a sidewalk with a bike, you would know that you can't just ride onto it. You will crash into the side. To get onto the sidewalk, you need to lift your front wheel. This isn't easy to get right, and to do it, you need some skills and some practice.

Important: Not all bikes are made to do jumps, manuals, hops, or even wheel lifts. If your bike doesn't have suspension, you don't get the bounce you need to lift up. And even some bikes that have suspension, like Enduro bikes, are not designed for jumping.

So make sure that if you do want to start doing lifts or jumps, you have a bike that will let you play.

Bend Your Arms

Get into the same position you get into when climbing a hill. Bend your elbows and bring them towards your ribs.

Use Your Hips

You probably think that if you want to lift your front wheel, it is all about pulling the handlebars, right? But with a manual, there is actually very little effort from your arms. If you keep your body in line with the bike like we have been teaching you, it is extremely difficult just to lift the front of the bike using your arms.

We have also been talking about how important it is to keep your body in the middle of the bike, so that you spread your weight evenly. But for a manual, this is the only time you have to move your weight unequally on the bike. If you don't take your weight off the front of the bike, it is going to be extremely difficult to lift the front.

Bend your Knees

If you are leaning all the way back with your bum, you will see that your bike will almost automatically start lifting in the front. Bending your knees will press more weight down the middle, and allow the bike to tip. But you have to do this in a controlled way; otherwise, you will just go all the way onto your back.

Stomp

The power to lift off the ground comes from the stomping movement on the bike. So, bend your knees and your elbows, and stomp on your pedals. As your bike comes up, shift your bum backward over the seat, so that the wheel lifts in the front.

The moment your front wheel starts lifting, bend your legs some more, and then move your hips forward a bit. You have to make sure that you move your weight back and forward on the seat at certain times to make sure the wheel lifts all the way back.

As the wheel starts to lift, you can let it go as high as you need to. But when you need it to go back down, you have to move your weight to the front of the seat again.

Back Wheel Lift

Now that you've gotten the hang of lifting your front wheel, start trying to lift your back wheel. The best way to do this is by standing tall with your legs and arms straight. Bend your legs and arms a little, and stomp on the pedals to make yourself bounce. As your bike bounces up, push your hips and shoulders forward, over your handlebars. Don't go too far forward, but just enough so your back wheel lifts off the ground. You will have to try and test this a few times to see how hard you have to stomp, and how far forward you have to lean before the wheel starts lifting.

Bunny Hops

So, if you've got the hang of the rear wheel lift and the front wheel lift, you are ready for the next step. Those are not easy skills to do, so if you can do one (or both), you are doing extremely well!

The next thing to do is a bunny hop. This is where you lift both wheels off the ground. This doesn't mean that both wheels are lifted at the same time. With a bunny hop, you first lift one wheel and then the other. That's why it was so important to first practice just lifting the back wheel, and then just the front wheel. You were getting ready to lift them right after each other.

Start with your speed. To do a hop, you don't want to be going fast. Go about as slow as walking speed.

1. Keep your chin up. No matter how you hop your bike, it is important to keep your chin up and heels dropped the entire time.
2. Go into the position you go into when you are on an uphill. Bend your elbows against your ribs, and bend toward your handlebar with your bum out.
3. Move your body and weight backward toward the back wheel. It helps if you push your bum back a little, and put the weight firmly in your hips and feet.
4. You now have to combine what you did with your front wheel and back wheel lifts.

5. To lift both wheels, you need some hop power, so you're going to have to stomp on your pedals again.

6. Bend your knees, stomp your pedals, and shift your bum back to lift the front wheel.

7. The moment your front wheel is in the air, scoop your legs forward and push your handlebars away from you. This will lift your back wheel in the air.

Jumps

Wait! Before you start trying to do jumps, it is so important that you first get the other skills right. Don't try and do jumps or wheelies until you have learned the basic skills. These jumps and wheelies can take months to practice and learn. Make sure you are completely comfortable on a bike, with all the other skills before you try doing jumps and wheelies.

And when you do try these tricks, always wear as much protective gear as possible. Make sure you are wearing your helmet correctly, and wear your kneepads and elbow pads if you have them.

These are not skills that you should just try anytime. You can get hurt, and nobody wants that.

Jumps will be slightly different than your bunny hops and your manual. With a jump, you won't be on flat ground. You will be going up a slight hill. So you will do a lot of the same things you did with your smaller jumps, but in a slightly different way.

Preparing for Take-Off

1. The first part of the jump is when you're still on the ground. Keep your basics in mind, push your heels down, keep your chin up, and bring your chest close to the handlebar.

2. Just like with the easier jumps, you want to stomp onto your pedals. The right term for this stomping movement is a preload, which means you are forcing your bike down so that it gives you a spring upwards.
3. It's all about timing. The time you preload, and the time you lift your wheel depends on where you are on the hill.
4. Just like with the other lifts, you want to focus on one wheel at a time.
5. If you have a dropper post, it is a good idea to lower it as you start riding toward a jump, so you have more room to move around on the bike.

Take-Off

6. Just before you are about to jump, press down onto the pedals and do a preload.
7. When your bike pops back from the preload, you have to push your handlebars away, and push all your weight onto your pedals.
8. It is very important that you push your handlebars away *before* your bike lifts off the ground. If you don't, the weight will go forward, and you can fall over your handlebars.

Landing

9. You are in the air! Getting your bike off the ground was the most difficult part. Now, all you have to do is land safely.
10. Remember we said that you should always look at where you want your bike to go? Well, look at where you want your bike to land. And point your bike that way too.
11. It is important to land with both wheels at the same time, so that you don't fall forward or backward.
12. As you start to land, you will see if you are leaning too far forward, or too far back. That way, you will be able to move so that your wheels land at the same time.

13. Straighten your arms and your legs as you get ready to land your bike. If you are bent too closely to your bike, you could lose control.

This is a lot of words, and a lot of things to remember. But the more times you read this and practice this, the more it will make sense.

As you do this over and over you will start to feel what you are doing wrong, and what works best. So the next time you do it, you will know to change your body a little bit to get higher or further. You will start to feel exactly where you need to preload, and when to change your weight, so that you have the perfect jump.

A lot of the mountain biking skills that you will learn are all about feeling what works, and going with what feels right. Just like with corners, berm, and switchbacks.

You will see that when you do the corner or the jumps, at first it will feel extremely strange. It is uncomfortable, and it feels strange to be in that position on the bike, especially if you are very used to sitting or standing on your bike just to ride normally.

It will feel wrong in the beginning, but that's okay. Just keep riding and keep practicing these tricks, and you will start to see that it becomes a lot better with time. As you start to do these more, you will become more comfortable, and get used to that position on the bike. And before you know it, you will become a jumping expert, moving your body in all kinds of ways while you are in the air.

Wheelie

A wheelie is almost like a manual, but there is one difference: the pedaling. When you are doing a manual, your wheel is usually just in the air for a few seconds, so you can get over the high ledge. But with a wheelie, your wheel stays in the air for as long as you want it, and you have to keep pedaling and moving to keep it there.

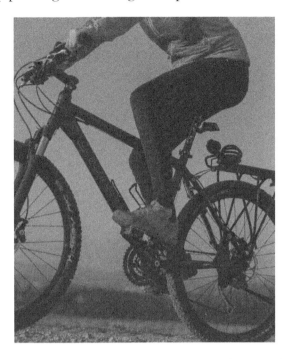

To do a wheelie, there are a few things you can do to make it easier to get it right.

1. Lower your seat if you have a dropper post. If you don't, just stay sitting on your saddle.
2. Change your gears so that you are in about the same gear you would use on the trails. This is a medium or slightly easier gear.
3. Get some movement on your bike, and just let it roll forward.
4. While sitting down, crouch over your handlebars so that the weight is in the front of your bike.
5. Turn your pedals so that they are at a 10:00 angle. This means that if your pedals were arms on a clock, they would be positioned so that your leading foot would show 10 o'clock. This is just so you have some power to pull up.
6. Pedal down, and at the same time, pull on your handlebars.

7. When you do this, lean back so that the wheel lifts, but don't flick back too quickly, or you might fall on your back. Keep pedaling, and stretch your arms out while you sit on the tip of your seat.

8. Just like with normal riding, make sure your fingers are on the brake. But when doing a wheelie, you will only be pushing your back brake.

9. You have to press the back brake softly the entire time, or you'll go too quickly. So, keep pedaling, and when you feel you are going too fast, brake softly.

10. Practice, practice, practice.

Most pro-cyclists can't do a wheelie. It is something that takes a special type of skill, and it takes a lot of time to perfect. Don't get frustrated and give up, because it does take time and a lot of practice. You have to get used to the feeling of the bike in the air. You also have to practice serious balance, since you will only be on one wheel. But the moment you start practicing and getting used to it, you will get it right in no time.

Chapter 7:

Tools and Kits to Always Carry

With You

Medical tools and safety tools that come in handy all the time.

When you are riding trails or long distances, you never know what can happen while you are on your bike. Your bike isn't break-proof, and there are so many things that can break, bend, flatten or fall off. So the best thing you can do is prepare yourself for any bike emergencies, so that you don't have to carry your bike all the way to the starting point. If you are riding three-hour trails, and something happens, you are going to have to push your bike all the way back. Believe me, it's not fun.

So make the effort to carry a few things with you that will help on the trails. These tools can be kept in a small pouch that you strap onto your seat. You can buy them from most mountain bike shops. Or, you can keep them in a small backpack with you. But just don't forget this backpack at home when you cycle. If you get a puncture on the trail and your puncture kit is in your backpack at home, you're going to be pretty upset with yourself.

Multi-Tool

A multi-tool is definitely the most important thing you can carry with you when you are on the trails. There are a few things on a multi-tool that can help you in different ways. There are also a few different types of multi-tools that have different parts in them, but these are the usually the types of tools on them:

- Hex key (also called an Allen key), which is used to turn bolts and screws that have a hexagon-shaped head. This key is used to change your seat post, or the levers on your handlebar.
- Torx heads, which are used to loosen and tighten another type of bolt. These bolts are usually around your disk brakes.
- Screwdriver
- A tire lever, which helps you get your tire off the rim if it needs to be fixed.
- Pliers or wire cutters

It is great to have a multi-tool with you if something happens on the trails. But don't try and change any part of your bike without the help of someone who has done it before. If you start loosening things in your bike that you don't know about, you can damage your bike. Even worse, you can get hurt if parts of your bike are loose.

Spare Tube

It is important to carry a spare tube with you so that you can fix your tire if something happens to it on the trail. A spare tube will work with both a tubeless and tubed wheel. The only difference will be how you fix it. Again, it is important that you make sure that someone helps you when working with these tools and spares. It is always better to have someone help you who has done it before, because it isn't the easiest thing to do.

Mini Pump

A mini pump is the best thing you can carry with you for a flat tire on the trails. It is small enough to fit in a small backpack. All you have to do is put it on our bike valve, and use your hands to pump your tire.

Puncture Repair Kit

Repair kits have everything you need if something happens to your tire, especially after you've used your spare tube. The best kit to have is the tubeless plug kit. There are basically only two things in the kit that will help you fix most punctures.

We will explain how you can fix certain problems on your bike, so that you know what to do. But as always, it is a good idea to get someone who has experience doing these things to help you . So if any of these issues happen while you are riding, try to get another rider to help you fix it.

Fixing a Punctured Tire

The first sign that you have a tire puncture is that you will have a flat tire. It is important not to ride on a flat tire because of the damage it can cause. If you have a tubeless tire and the hole is very small, the sealant inside your tire will seal the hole immediately.

You should first pump the tire with your mini-pump and see if the tire stays pumped. If it doesn't, and you can see it going flat again, you probably have a puncture.

Look at the tire for anything that could have caused the puncture. Look for any thorns, glass, sticks, or nails. It is important to take this out before you fix the tire. If you don't, the thorn, glass, or nail will just damage it again.

To fix a puncture, the first step is to peel the plug out of the paper. You will see the plug looks like long, thin strips of clay. Pull off a strip of the plug and pull it through the tool. It is the same as threading thread through a needle.

Once the plug is halfway through the 'needle,' fold the two points together.

Now you have to stick this needle into the hold. Stick it in all the way, but let the plug piece hang out.

As you pull the tool out of the hole, the plug will stay behind, and hang out of the hole.

If there is a long piece hanging out, just cut it shorter. But it is normal for it to hang out the hole. You can leave it like this each time you ride, and don't need to replace the tire. This plug basically becomes part of your tire forever.

Chain Lube

It is important to always keep your chain lubed, to prevent the metal from grinding against the other metal while you are riding. In the next chapter, we explain how to take care of your bike well. One of the things is to ensure your chain is always lubed. If you ride long distances, keep chain lube with you so you can always add some to the chain if necessary.

Tire Lever

Some multi-tools add a tire lever, which you use to take your tire off the rim so that you can replace or fix it. It is better to carry a separate tire lever with you because the multi-tool ones are sometimes too small, and don't work as well.

Derailleur Hanger

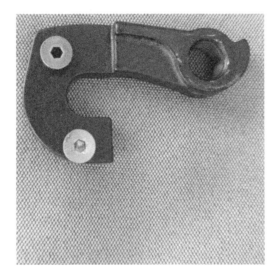

A derailleur hanger is a part of the back of your bike and holds a few important parts of your bike together. It goes onto your bike frame, and was designed to bend and break in a way that prevents damage to your frame. The only problem is that when this breaks, you will not be able to keep riding. There is no way you would be able to change gears and take on a trail.

It is important that you carry a spare with you that is designed for your specific brand and bike make. Each derailleur is different depending on the bike and model. So you won't be able to use someone else's derailleur if yours breaks on a trail. You will need to carry your own spare.

Master Link

When you look at your chain, you will see that it is made of hundreds of individual links that clip into each other. Sometimes, when you are riding down certain trails, your chain can get caught or damaged, and one of these links can break.

When that happens, you won't be able to ride your bike at all, and will need to walk home. But if you have some tools with you, you can fix and replace these links, and keep on riding.

A master link is a type of link that connects the links that are already on your bike. What's great about having a master link on your bike is that you can open and close this link, and take your chain off if you need to give it a deep clean.

Sunscreen

Having a small bottle of sunscreen with you at all times is really important, especially if you are going to ride often and ride far. Sunlight is great, and you need vitamin D. But spending hours and hours in the sun without protection only causes trouble.

Before going on a ride, put sunscreen on all the parts of your body that are exposed to the sun. Remember the parts behind your neck, over your ears, and especially on your calves. As you ride and sweat on the trails, just stop for a drink of water after a while, and add some more sunscreen.

Zip Ties and Duct Tape

Zip ties and duct tape are things that not enough people talk about. They are two of the most useful things to carry with you, and will help with many different things.

If anything on your bike is loose or shaky, zip ties or duct tape will help you keep everything together long enough for you to get off the trails, and have it fixed.

If there is an injury and you need to keep the bandage in place, duct tape helps for that too. If your shoe buckle or helmet breaks somewhere, duct tape is your friend!

Trust us on this, and carry these with you in your bag. You don't have to carry a whole roll of duct tape with you. You can just roll off a long piece (but roll it with the sticky piece outside) and put that in your bag.

Co2 Bomb and Inflator (Optional)

A Co2 bomb is a small metal container that you can carry around with you if you need an emergency tire pump. Many riders will carry this instead of a mini-pump, so we will explain how to use it. But as a beginner, don't carry around a bomb, and use the mini-pump instead.

These bombs are great for three main uses:

- Your tire is flat while riding on a trail
- You got a puncture on the trail, and need to pump your tire after fixing the puncture
- You had to change the tire and pump it up afterward

VERY IMPORTANT: These Co2 bombs are extremely dangerous to handle without a glove. Because of the metal that holds the gas inside, the metal gets so cold when you use the bomb that it can burn your skin when you use it without a glove.

So you can either get yourself a bomb-glove, which you put around the metal and carry with you. Or you have to make sure you are wearing a glove when you use the bomb. If you don't have a bomb-glove or hand-glove when using it, use a cloth to hold it. But you should never, ever hold the metal while using it.

With the bomb, you also have to carry around an inflator. This adaptor is used so that you can transfer the gas from the bomb into your tire. It screws onto your bomb, which you can then turn into your tire valve.

Emergency Kit

If something happens while you are on the trails, you don't want to have to wait until you're home before you start treating the injury. If you have any scrapes or open cuts, your water bottles are great to rinse them off immediately. But sometimes you have to carry more with you. In the next chapter, we will take a look at exactly what you need for emergencies.

Basic Emergency Kit to Have

It's not fun to think about, but the reality is that mountain-biking can be a dangerous sport. If you aren't careful, you can get seriously hurt. And sometimes, even when you are extremely careful, you can *still* get hurt.

But this is true for many other sports, and a lot of things in life. Some fun things are also dangerous. But you can't avoid doing them because you might get hurt. What you can do, though, is prepare for when something happens, and take care of it.

Some shops sell special mountain bike emergency kits that you can just clip onto your backpack. But if you want to carry just a few basic things with you, this is what we suggest.

Different-shaped Bandaid

In most cases, when you fall, you will just scrape a part of your arm or leg, and you need nothing else than a bandaid. So make sure you carry some big and small ones, and ones in different shapes. These shapes and sizes will help you put a bandaid on any part of your body, on a wound of any size.

Bandages and Gauzes

Sometimes, if it is a serious injury, bandaids are not going to be big enough. So keep bandages and gauzes for if you have a big wound that you have to cover. You can also just keep gauzes in your bag with duct tape. This means you can use duct tape instead to keep the gauze in place.

Anti-Bacterial Wipes

You can wait until you get home before cleaning the wounds properly. But we suggest keeping a few anti-bacterial wipes with you to clean off any scrapes, cuts, or bigger wounds. You don't want to get an infection anywhere, so these wipes will keep things clean until you have space to clean everything well.

Emergency Contact Number

Also, it's always a good idea to keep an emergency number with you every time you ride. Some riders stick the number to their bikes, or tie it around their arms. You can keep these numbers on your phone too, but it will be difficult for someone else to access your phone if you have a password. Or, if you have fallen and broken your phone, you can see why that would be a problem.

So, always keep a number on you. Even if you remember the number, write it down and keep it with you. Sometimes riders who fall go into shock, and can't remember the number. So, better be safe and keep it on paper.

Since we are talking about emergency numbers, the other thing to keep with you is a list of emergency services around you. If you are riding alone and need the local ambulance, it is a good idea to write down their number too. Some areas also have a number for the local animal control unit, which helps you if you have a snake bite.

Your Own Medication

If you have serious medical conditions that need certain medicine, make sure you remember to take that with you on the ride. If you need things like an asthma inhaler, EpiPen, or insulin for diabetes, always keep extras in your backpack!

Notes for Broken Bones

For more serious injuries, like a broken bone, many riders carry something called a splint. It is just a hard object that keeps your arm or leg in place so that you don't move it with your broken bone. Other riders suggest that if you fall and break something, you should just use a stick instead of a splint.

If you are comfortable with adding something else to your bike when riding, take a splint with you. But when you are working with a broken bone, you will definitely need some help keeping the arm or leg in place, and wrapping it against the splint or stick.

Other Things You Can Carry

Anti-bacterial wipes, gauzes, and bandaids are the most important things to have with you at all times. Of course, this includes your duct tape and zip ties, since they hold many things in place. But if you have space in your bag, here are a few ideas about other tools to carry with you on the trails.

Whistle: if you ever ride alone and something happens to you, a whistle is great to carry with you on the bike, so you can get the attention of fellow riders for help.

Money: If you ever have to ride somewhere to fix your bike, you can pay for the repair with the cash you carry.

Chapter 8:

How to Take Care of Your Bike

(and yourself)

Taking care of yourself and your bike so you can continue enjoying the sport

Your bike is tough. It can handle rocky roads, trails, jumps, falls, and long hours on the road. But even though it is that tough, you still need to take care of it, especially after those hard rides.

So there are ways you can look after your bike to make sure it lasts long, and doesn't need as many services and fixes. Here is what you should do to keep your bike in perfect condition.

Washing Your Bike

Washing your bike isn't just about making it look nice. Washing your bike is one of the most important things to do to prevent damage.

When you ride through sandy or muddy areas, those tiny sand pieces sit in all the holes and gaps on your bike. And as you ride your bike, the sand scratches against all the metal pieces and seriously damages it. Here's what you need to clean your bike:

- High-pressure hose
- Bike wash
- Chain wash
- Metal brush

- Dry Cloth
- Chain lube

1. The best thing to do is to wash your bike with high pressure, like through a hose. Make sure you get in between all the moving parts. Move your pedal forward, and lift your seat so you can get water into all those gaps.
2. The water is not enough, though. Get yourself a special bike wash soap that is designed to clean your bike the way it needs to be cleaned. Spray your entire bike with this bike wash. Don't be afraid to make it really soapy.
3. You should also get yourself a special soap made for your chain and cassette. This soap is used to take the grease off your chain, so be careful not to spray it on any other part of your bike, except the chain and cassette.
4. Use the metal brush to brush the chain. You should brush it, turn your pedal so that the chain moves, and brush again. You really want to get in between all those gaps.
5. Use the pressure hose to rinse off all the soap and dry it off with a cloth.
6. Now that you've taken off the grease and lube from the chain, you have to replace it. So make sure you put some lube on the chain. Turn the pedals as you do this so that you get lube on the whole chain.

Lubing the Chain

In the previous chapter, we have said that you should keep lube on the trail with you. And now you know you should also put lube on after you've washed it.

But what is lube used for and how often should you use it?

The lube on your chain is to prevent the rubbing of metal on metal from damaging your bike. So the lube lets the chain run from the crankset to the cassette through all the gears, without grinding against the metal.

It is best to lube your chain for every two or three rides. You don't have to do too much, or they might get too slippery. But just a quick squeeze on the chain is fine.

Keeping Your Tire Pressure Up

In the first part of the book you learned exactly how to pump the tires, and what they should be on. It is important to check your tire pressure before every ride. If your tires are too flat, you can get injured because your tire doesn't have enough traction. But other than that, a flat wheel can also hurt the bike rim. And the bike rim is not cheap to replace, so don't take a chance by not checking it.

Taking Care of Yourself

Now that you know how to take care of your bike before a ride, have you ever thought about how to take care of yourself? Just like your mountain bike takes a lot of strain when riding those trails, your body also takes strain. Riding a bike uses muscles in all parts of your body. And if it is something your body isn't used to, you will start to feel stiff and sore a lot. It is so important to take care of your body, inside and outside, so that you can continue enjoying the sport.

As a rider, you have to make sure you work on the muscles you use during riding. You also have to make sure these muscles get stretched properly.On top of that, you have to make sure that you are eating and drinking all the right foods to help your muscles recover. If you don't get the right nutrients into your body, you are going to be tired all the time, and you'll take longer to recover after a ride.

Here is what we suggest beginners do to take care of their bodies.

Strengthen Your Cycling Muscles

Did you know that if you have weak stomach muscles you have less balance and control on your bike? Yeah, that's crazy to think about. As a rider, you think your legs do all the work. They're the ones pedaling and moving your bike, right?

Well, your legs do a lot of the work. But keeping your body upright also means you have to have strong arms. And for balance, your core muscles need to be strong. If your aim is to be a really good cyclist, we suggest you do some exercises when you're not on the bike, so that you become better when you're on the bike.

Planks

Planks are a great workout to strengthen your arms and core at the same time. To start, you have to lie flat on your stomach with your hands right underneath your armpits. Push yourself off the ground, and hold your body in a plank position on your toes.

Make sure you pull in your stomach muscles, and keep your back straight. Don't stick your bum in the air. Hold this position for as long as you can, and really try to push yourself. When you can't hold it anymore, lie down for about ten seconds. Try it again after that, and do this three or four times. If you want, you can also time yourself, and see how long you could hold the position each time. So, as you practice this, after a few days and week, you will be able to see how much stronger you get, and how much longer you can hold the position.

If it is too difficult to do this position, first try doing it on your elbows. Put your forearms on the ground instead of holding your body up with your hands. Just remember to keep a straight back, and try to look forward.

PushUps

Another great workout to do to strengthen your cycling muscles is pushups. The same muscles you use when doing a pushup are the muscles you use when keeping yourself upright, and moving your bike around.

There are many different types of pushups you can do, depending on your strength.

If you have no strength in your arms, try doing wall pushups. Stand away from the wall and put your hands flat against the wall. Make sure you stand away far enough so that you straighten your arms. Then, lean your body forward like you would with a normal pushup.

Your thumbs should be by your armpits when you do this movement. And when you lean towards the wall, don't let your elbows stick out to the side. Make sure they stay against your ribs with each movement. Do about ten of these to start with, take about a 30-second break, and then do it two more times.

If you have some strength in your arms, you can try doing pushups on the floor. The position is just like the plank position one. If you are still not too strong, you can do the pushup from your knees. When you get stronger, you can do it from your toes.

Squats

Just because you need to make sure your arms and core are strong doesn't mean you should forget about your legs. Your legs do most of the work, so the stronger you make them when you are not cycling, the easier it will be when you do cycle.

When doing a squat, the muscles you work include your quads, glutes, hamstrings, and knees. These are all the muscles that work when you cycle too.

To do a squat, stand with your legs shoulder-distance apart. Your feet should be pointing out just a little bit. Keep your core tight, and slowly go into a sitting position. The lower you go the better, and you should try to touch the ground with your bum every time. Make sure you check that your knees are not going past your toes. You should stick your bum out, and not let your knees go too far forward. If your knees go forward, you are doing it wrong, and can hurt your knees if you keep doing squats this way.

Start by doing ten squats. Take about a 30-second break and do that again two or three times. The stronger you get, the more you will be able to do at a time. The next time, try doing twenty, thirty, forty, or fifty at a time.

Kettlebell Swings

You will not believe how good kettlebell swings are for your body, especially if you are trying to become a stronger cyclist. The movement is perfect for staying on the bike longer without getting tired. It also helps to strengthen your *pedal stroke,* which means you have more power when you pedal.

To do this exercise, choose a comfortable kettlebell weight. Then, stand with your legs shoulder-width apart, and bend your knees a little. Hold the kettlebell with both hands in front of you. In one movement, swing the kettlebell up to your chest while keeping your arms straight the entire time. When you want to let it fall back down, don't just let it swing freely. Use your strength to lower it back to the starting position slowly.

With each of these movements, use your hips to help you swing. When the kettlebell comes up, swing your hips forward. When you slowly lower it, push your hips back.

Do fifteen of these, and then take a one-minute break. Then do it again. If you can, do this three or four times each day.

Burpees

Everyone loves a good burpee, right? Burpees are another full-body workout that will help you strengthen all the parts needed for the bike. Since there are a few different movements, you are working a ton of different muscle groups.

Separate your feet shoulder-distance apart, bend your legs, and put your hands on the floor. Then, jump up a little and straighten your legs out behind you, so that you are on your toes in a plank position. If you can, do a pushup. If you can't, leave out the pushup.

From here, bring your legs back into your starting position, and jump into the air. You will be jumping back and forth, up and down. When you are done with your jump, reach down and put your hands on the ground again, so you can straighten your legs and repeat all of that.

Try starting with ten of these burpees. Rest for a minute, and then repeat them three or four times. When you start doing this often, you will start seeing a huge difference in your strength and fitness on your bike.

Stretch Your Muscles

If you aren't stretching after each workout and after each cycle, you are going to be stiff and sore for a lot longer than necessary. Also, what a lot of people don't realize is that because cycling is the same movement over and over again, there is a lot of tension in the muscles and joints.

By stretching and having better flexibility, your muscles and bones will be healthier and work better.

To start off stretching, try these stretches made for cyclists, and do them right after a cycle. You will undo any strain you put on your body.

Hips

You can probably guess why your hips get tight after a cycle. The way you sit, and the muscles you use, all come from your hips. A lot of tightness after a ride will come from your hips, which you can prevent from happening by stretching.

To stretch your hips, stand on your knees. Then, lift one leg and put it in front of you with your toes pointing forward. If you have ever done a runner's lunge, this stretch is similar. But the knee that you are standing on stays beneath your hip.

Put your hands on the foot that is forward, and press your leg forward using your hands. You will feel a stretch in the opposite hip and front of the leg. Do this for about ten seconds on each side five times.

Hamstrings

A lot of your cycling power comes from the back of your legs. The pedaling motion uses a lot of your calf and hamstring muscles. So, stretching is extremely important. Not only is it good to prevent yourself from being stiff in the morning, but it also helps the muscles grow and stretch into a long muscle. With some exercises, the muscles in your body become short, but by stretching them you stretch out the muscle, and help it to develop into a long, healthy muscle.

Stand on your knees again, and put your one foot forward as far as you can go. You will have to put your heel to the ground, and point your toes to the sky. Sit backward, but keep your back tall. The further you go back, the more you will feel the stretch in the back of your leg.

Don't make it painful for yourself. Just sit back until you can feel the stretch in the back of your leg.

Keep this up for about twenty seconds, then swap legs.

Glutes

Your bum muscles are on the saddle most of the time, but that doesn't mean they aren't working. Stretching your glutes will also give you better movement around your hips, which will make your riding better too.

So, to stretch your glutes, lay down flat on your back with your legs straight up. Bend one leg, and put that foot on the other knee. Your legs will look like a number 4. Then, hold your straight leg behind your knee, and put that leg towards your chest.

You will feel that there is a stretch in the leg that is bent. Do this for 30 seconds, and switch legs.

Calves

If you start cycling a lot, you will start to see a lot of muscle start to form in your calves. That's because your calves do a lot of the pedaling work, which also means they need some good stretching.

To stretch your calves, stand on your hands and knees with your feet flat on the ground. Your legs don't have to be close to your body. The shape of your body will look more like a triangle. You can walk your feet a little closer to your hands until your calves really start pulling, and you feel you are quite stiff.

That's when you should bend one knee and push the other foot's heel towards the ground. The point is to feel the pull and stretch in the back of your straight leg's calf and leg. Do this for about 10 seconds, and then bend that leg and straighten the other one. You can repeat this about three or four times.

Quads

The fronts of your legs also need some stretching, because they work just as hard as the rest of your leg.

To stretch your quads, stand up straight next to a wall and bend your legs. Using your hand, bend that foot towards your bum, until you feel the stretch at the front of your leg. You can use your other hand to hold onto the wall for balance.

You can do this for about 30 seconds, then switch legs.

What to Eat and Drink When Cycling

What you eat, when you eat, and what you drink can all affect how you ride. It also affects how you feel after a ride, and how long you take to recover.

It is important to know that there are a few tricks to eating and drinking that will help your body use the right nutrients and give you energy.

Not only is it important to eat and drink certain things while you are cycling, but there are things you have to eat and drink before and afterward, since your body is constantly working and burning calories.

What to Eat Before a Ride

You have to eat something before you go for a ride so that you have the fuel, and give your body some energy to work with. You are filling up on food that helps fill up on your glycogen levels (which basically means you are putting fuel in your tank.) The food you want to eat before a ride is mainly carbohydrates and protein, which is a great source of fuel for your tank. You should try and eat about an hour before you go for a ride.

Oatmeal: If you are going for a cycle in the morning, an oatmeal breakfast is a perfect way to get in your protein and carb fuel. You can add things like peanut butter, chia seeds, and bananas, which are all great sources of protein that will help you fill up.

Bread: Bread is another great option for before a ride. But make sure you get low-GI bread, which means it releases energy slowly. So that means no white bread. You can add any type of protein to this, like eggs or peanut butter. That makes a great combination of protein and carbs before a ride.

What to Eat and Drink During a Ride

What you eat and drink during a ride depends on how long your ride will be. If you are just riding for an hour or two, make sure you drink plenty of water. But if you are riding for two or three hours, you should get yourself a sports drink.

These sports drinks have lots of electrolytes, which is very important for you and your body. You can also carry an energy bar which has carbs, protein, and fat with you. A banana and some nuts are also great snacks for rides. And, of course, you want to drink as much water as you can.

What to Eat and Drink After a Ride

After you had such a long ride, you are going to have to eat a good meal with protein, fat, and carbs. Try to eat at least one hour after a ride so that you can help your body recover after all the work it did. And don't forget to drink water, even after a ride. You did a lot of sweating on your bike, and should keep drinking water to stay hydrated.

Conclusion

There are a lot of things to remember about how to handle your bike, how to sit, and what to do with your gears and brakes. But the most important thing to remember, each time you get on a bike, is to have fun.

Remember, the reason you're learning how to ride a mountain bike is so that you can enjoy all the fun it brings! There is so much excitement in riding new trails, learning new skills, and being outdoors.

You're going to have a lot of days where you are frustrated. Not everything you try you will get right the first few times. But don't forget the number one rule: *have fun*.

Mountain bikes are a great place to learn patience. They also teach you not to be too hard on yourself, and let yourself make mistakes. But most importantly, learning to ride a mountain bike teaches you that if you really want something, you have to keep going, keep practicing and keep struggling. If you really want it, you will keep on, even on the days that it feels like you want to give up.

Because I promise, the day you do a jump, or a switchback, or a get to the top of the hill you never thought you could get up, you are going to feel crazy proud of yourself. And all the struggles, tears, and falls you had will be worth it when you finally get it right.

Inspiring Riders

If you want some more inspiration and ideas for mountain bike riders who have gone through what you are going through and have done amazing things, have a look at these YouTubers:

Rachel Atherton is a professional downhill mountain biker, and she is incredible on her bike. She is a six-time World Champion, six-time World Cup Champion, and she has 40 individual World Cup wins. If you want to learn about downhilling, she is the person you should watch for motivation and inspiration.

Greg Minnaar doesn't have his own channel, but the videos of him on YouTube will definitely inspire you. He is excellent at explaining certain skills and tricks and, of course, shows us how he does amazing things on his bike.

Aaron Gwin has an amazing channel that talks about everything mountain biking. He shows great workouts, does skill videos, and also has crazy go-pro footage of him on some scary trails.

Danny MacAskill is a hardcore rider, doing stunts, tricks, and rides that seem impossible. He loves using his bike to do tricks and stunts, and is an expert at jumps and bunny hops. So if you want to learn more about that, Danny is the perfect guy to watch.

Tracy Moseley is another expert female rider who has incredible videos. She doesn't have her own channel, but YouTube is filled with videos of her doing outstanding skills videos. She teaches everything from wheelies to climbing.

When you watch these videos, don't forget that each one of these riders started out as a beginner. They didn't just get on a bike one day and jump, wheelie, or win World Championships. They all started somewhere, unsure and unskilled. But what got them to their level of riding was practice, and their willingness never to give up. Use them as motivation to see how far you can go if you just keep trying.

And always remember to keep your chin up and *just keep pedaling.*

References

A Perfect MTB Rear Wheel Lift. (n.d.). Learn.ryanleech.com. https://learn.ryanleech.com/blog/perfect-mtb-rear-wheel-lift

Andrews, E. (2021 February 18). *The Bicycle's Bumpy History*. HISTORY. https://www.history.com/news/bicycle-history-invention#:~:text=A%20German%20baron%20named%20Karl

Ballin, P. (2021 November 17). *Trail Bike VS Enduro Bike | Which Is Better?* Bike Faff. Bike Faff. https://bikefaff.com/trail-bike-vs-enduro-bike/

Barber, J. (2018 January 11). *How to Set Your Mountain Bike Seat Height... And Why It's So Important*. Singletracks Mountain Bike News. https://www.singletracks.com/mtb-gear/set-mountain-bike-seat-height-important/

Bayer, C. (2015 January 9). *How to Set up your Brake Levers perfectly*. ENDURO Mountainbike Magazine. https://enduro-mtb.com/en/how-to-set-up-your-brake-levers-perfectly/

Bennett, R. (2018 January 17). *Hardtail versus full suspension bikes*. Red Bull. https://www.redbull.com/se-en/hardtail-versus-full-suspension-mtb-bikes

Bennett, R. (2021 January 19). *6 top tips to improve your uphill riding*. Red Bull. https://www.redbull.com/za-en/top-tips-to-improve-your-mtb-climbing

Bennett, R. (2021 February 16). *5 top tips for nailing a MTB manual*. Red Bull. https://www.redbull.com/us-en/how-to-do-a-mountain-bike-manual

BETD Components: How to find the best MTB crankset for you. (2018 September 4). BETD. https://www.mountainbikecomponents.co.uk/cranksets/determining-the-best-mtb-crank-set-for-you/

Bezdek, N., & Lodge, G. (2020 February 28). *The Beginner's Guide to Shifting Gears on a Bike.* Bicycling. https://www.bicycling.com/training/a20004265/how-to-shift/

Brayton, D. (2021 August 6). *BMX Bike Vs Mountain Bike – Which One Right For You?* Electricalwheel.com. https://electricalwheel.com/bmx-bike-vs-mountain-bike/

Choosing the Best Mountain Bike Helmet. (2019 May 20). Bicycle Warehouse. https://bicyclewarehouse.com/blogs/news/best-mountain-bike-helmets

cyclingmag. (2020 August 9). *Beginner's guide to every type of mountain bike.* Canadian Cycling Magazine. https://cyclingmagazine.ca/mtb/beginners-guide-mountain-bike-types/

Evans, A. (2020 April 17). *Mountain bike wheel sizes: 26in, 650b and 29in explained.* BikeRadar. https://www.bikeradar.com/mtb/mountain-bike-wheel-sizes-26in-650b-and-29in-explained/

Fiske, B. (2010 April 30). *Basics Of Better Balance.* Bicycling. https://www.bicycling.com/training/a20009567/mountain-biking-tips-how-to-improve-balance/

Hinchliffe, S. (2016 January 12). *Bike Fit for MTB - Mountain Biking Australia magazine.* Www.mtbiking.com.au. https://www.mtbiking.com.au/how-to/bike-tech/cockpit-setup

How to Bunny Hop - Mountain Bike | Liv Cycling Official site. (2022). Liv-Cycling.com. https://www.liv-cycling.com/global/campaigns/how-to-bunny-hop-on-a-mountain-bike/19043

How to Choose a Mountain Bike: Buyer's Guide & Bike Types | evo. (2019). Evo.com. https://www.evo.com/guides/how-to-choose-mountain-bike

How to Choose Mountain Bike Pedals - Flats & Clipless | evo. (2022). Evo.com. https://www.evo.com/guides/how-to-choose-mountain-bike-pedals

How To Maintain Your Mountain Bike. (2016 December 18). Mantel. https://www.mantel.com/blog/en/how-to-maintain-your-mountain-bike

How to Wheelie on a Mountain Bike | Liv Cycling Official site. (2022). Liv-Cycling.com. https://www.liv-cycling.com/global/campaigns/how-to-wheelie-on-a-mountain-bike/23878

Hutchison, P. (n.d.). *Proper Foot Placement on a Bike Pedal.* LIVESTRONG.COM. https://www.livestrong.com/article/401973-proper-foot-placement-on-a-bike-pedal/

Jeff. (2015 October 16). *Mountain Bike Size...* Bicycle Guider - Bikes, Bike Reviews, Cycling Advice, Best Picks | Mountain, Road, Hybrid Bikes; Bicycle Guider. https://www.bicycle-guider.com/mountain-bike-size-chart/

Jonsson, H. (2021 April 5). *Why You Only Need One Jump to Become Amazing at Jumping.* Red Bull. https://www.redbull.com/se-en/how-to-become-good-at-mtb-jumping

Mateo, A. (2022 January 14). *These 6 Post-Ride Stretches Will Ease Soreness and Prevent Injury.* Bicycling. https://www.bicycling.com/training/a27683173/best-stretches/

MBR. (2019 November 12). *How to get better at cornering a mountain bike.* MBR. https://www.mbr.co.uk/news/how-to-corner-mountain-bike-347805

Milway, A. (2018 August 29). *Just how do downhill and enduro compare as racing disciplines?* Red Bull. https://www.redbull.com/za-en/mtb-downhill-vs-enduro

Milway, A. (2021 March 23). *5 simple ways to improve your mountain bike riding technique.* Red Bull. https://www.redbull.com/za-en/how-to-improve-your-mtb-technique

Mountain Bike Suspension Basics | Jenson USA. (n.d.). www.jensonusa.com. https://www.jensonusa.com/articles/mountain-bike-suspension-101#:~:text=Suspension%20is%20the%20nervous%20system

Mountain biking techniques - mounting and dismounting. (2022). Timeoutdoors.com. https://www.timeoutdoors.com/expert-advice/cycling/mountain-biking/mountain-biking-techniques-mounting-dismountin

Mountain Biking: How to Ride Berms. (n.d.). REI. https://www.rei.com/learn/expert-advice/mountain-biking-berms.html

MTB TIRE PRESSURE: EVERYTHING YOU NEED TO KNOW. (2017 November 24). Full Speed Ahead. https://www.fullspeedahead.com/en/technology/mtb-tire-pressure-everything-you-need-to-know#:~:text=Typical%20mountain%20bike%20pressures%20Orange

Paul, M. (2015 October 7). *50 Essential Items to Keep in your MTB Emergency Kits.* Singletracks Mountain Bike News. https://www.singletracks.com/uncategorized/50-essential-items-to-keep-in-your-mtb-emergency-kits/

published, R. S. (2021 August 3). *How to ride switchbacks: Take on tight corners with confidence.* Bike Perfect. https://www.bikeperfect.com/features/how-to-ride-switchbacks-take-on-tight-corners-with-confidence

Reed, E. (2021 August 24). *The 10 mountain bike accessories every beginner needs before hitting the trails.* Insider. https://www.insider.com/guides/health/fitness/best-mountain-biking-gear-for-beginners

Reed, Z. (2019 June 4). *The Complete Beginner's Guide To Mountain Bike Gears | Mountain Treads.* Mountain Treads. https://mountaintreads.com/guide-to-mountain-bike-gears/

Rome, D. (2016 September 22). *6 essential tools that every mountain biker should own.* BikeRadar. https://www.bikeradar.com/features/6-essential-tools-that-every-mountain-biker-should-own/

Ruben, A. (2018 December 10). *Differences Between a Mountain Bike and a Road Bike.* Bikinguniverse. https://www.bikinguniverse.com/differences-between-a-mountain-bike-and-a-road-bike/

What are the differences between eMTBs and standard Mountain Bikes? (2019 November 13). Pedal Cover. https://pedalcover.co.uk/cycle-blog/mountain-bike-vs-emtb#:~:text=How%20does%20an%20eMTB%20differ

What are the Parts of a Mountain Bike?» NTX Trails. (2018 September 19). NTX Trails. https://ntxtrails.com/parts-of-a-mountain-bike/

wheretheroadforks, A. (2021 February 14). *1X Vs 2X Drivetrain: Pros and Cons.* Where the Road Forks. https://wheretheroadforks.com/1x-vs-2x-drivetrain-pros-and-cons/

Why Mountain Bikers Should Wear Goggles. (2016 July 20). Demilked. https://www.demilked.com/why-mountain-bikers-should-wear-goggles/

Yare, A., Glass, A., Jonsson, H., & Roberts, D. (2021 January 18). *9 strength exercises that will make you a better cyclist.* Red Bull. https://www.redbull.com/za-en/cycling-strength-exercises-gym

Image References

Close Up of Bike Pedal · Free Stock Photo. (2016 November 2). Pexels. [Image] https://www.pexels.com/photo/close-up-of-bike-pedal-2801964/

gray chain photo – Free Grey Image on Unsplash. (2019 June 17). Unsplash. [Image] https://unsplash.com/photos/nJE9I1aKKvM

Kemp, P. (2021). *Derailleur Hanger.*

Kemp, P. (2022). *Switchbacks.*

man riding bicycle photo – Free Cuyuna lakes trails Image on Unsplash. (2019 July 11). Unsplash. https://unsplash.com/photos/Ep7llSmzHmQ

man riding mountain bike on hill under cloudy skies photo – Free Vladivostok Image on Unsplash. (2018 June 26). Unsplash. https://unsplash.com/photos/rNhbTQFEa-k

200+ Best Mountain Bike Photos · 100% Free Download · Pexels Stock Photos. (n.d.). Pexels. Retrieved March 13, 2022, from https://www.pexels.com/photo/black-and-green-bicycle-on-brown-dirt-93801/

Made in United States
North Haven, CT
24 July 2023

39458240R00068